SpringerBriefs in Public Health

SpringerBriefs in Public Health present concise summaries of cutting-edge research and practical applications from across the entire field of public health, with contributions from medicine, bioethics, health economics, public policy, biostatistics, and sociology.

The focus of the series is to highlight current topics in public health of interest to a global audience, including health care policy; social determinants of health; health issues in developing countries; new research methods; chronic and infectious disease epidemics; and innovative health interventions.

Featuring compact volumes of 55 to 125 pages, the series covers a range of content from professional to academic. Possible volumes in the series may consist of timely reports of state-of-the art analytical techniques, reports from the field, snapshots of hot and/or emerging topics, literature reviews, and in-depth case studies. Both solicited and unsolicited manuscripts are considered for publication in this series.

Briefs are published as part of Springer's eBook collection, with millions of users worldwide. In addition, Briefs are available for individual print and electronic purchase.

Briefs are characterized by fast, global electronic dissemination, standard publishing contracts, easy-to-use manuscript preparation and formatting guidelines, and expedited production schedules. We aim for publication 8–12 weeks after acceptance.

Germán Velásquez

Negotiating Global Health Policies

Tensions and Dilemmas

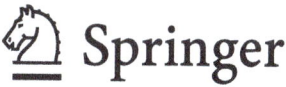 Springer

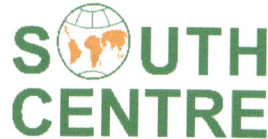

Germán Velásquez
Policy and Health South Centre
Geneva, Switzerland

ISSN 2192-3698   ISSN 2192-3701   (electronic)
SpringerBriefs in Public Health
ISBN 978-3-031-99846-1   ISBN 978-3-031-99847-8   (eBook)
https://doi.org/10.1007/978-3-031-99847-8

This Springer imprint is published by the registered company Springer Nature Switzerland AG
The registered company address is: Gewerbestrasse 11, 6330 Cham, Switzerland

If disposing of this product, please recycle the paper.

Acknowledgements

The author expresses his gratitude to Ms. Caroline Ngome Eneme for coordinating the publication process.

Contents

1	**Introduction**.	1
	References.	3
2	**Current Challenges and Possible Future Scenarios for Global Health**.	5
	2.1 Introduction.	5
	2.2 The World Bank and the International Monetary Fund.	7
	2.2.1 World Bank Intermediate Prevention, Preparedness and Response Fund.	8
	2.2.2 Goals and Roles of the World Bank FIF.	9
	2.2.3 Comments and Reactions to World Bank Reports on the FIF	9
	2.3 G7 - G20 - BRICS.	11
	2.4 The Group of 77 and China.	14
	2.5 The Non-Aligned Movement	15
	2.6 Philanthropy's Foray into Global Health.	16
	2.7 Public–Private Partnerships in Global Healthcare.	17
	2.8 New Concepts: Health Security, Universal Health Coverage	18
	2.9 The Role of Sustainable Development Objectives	19
	2.10 Conclusions: Three Possible Scenarios for the Future of Global Health	20
	2.10.1 Extension of the Current Status Quo	20
	2.10.2 Global Health in the Hands of the Private Sector?.	21
	2.10.3 Regional Solutions	21
	References.	22
3	**The Origins and Purpose of Global Health Financing**	25
	3.1 Introduction.	25
	3.2 Context	26
	3.3 Original WHO Funding Model (1948–1998)	27
	3.4 Funding of WHO Regional Offices.	28

3.4.1   The Unique Case of the Americas Regional Office:
         Mixed Funding 28
3.5   Kofi Annan's Global Compact at the United Nations 28
3.6   Progressive Privatization of the WHO: Increasing Reliance
       on Private, Philanthropic and Voluntary Public Contributions
       Beyond the Core Budge 30
3.7   Official Development Assistance for Health.................. 32
3.8   The Establishment of Parallel Organizations in the Health Sector .. 33
       3.8.1   UNAIDS 1996 34
       3.8.2   From the Expanded Programme on Immunization
                to the GAVI Partnership 34
       3.8.3   The Global Fund to Fight AIDS, Tuberculosis and
                Malaria 35
       3.8.4   Unitaid 36
       3.8.5   The Medicines Patent Pool...................... 37
       3.8.6   Coalition for Epidemic Preparedness Innovations
                (CEPI)... 38
       3.8.7   COVAX: 2021................................. 38
       3.8.8   The "WHO Foundation".......................... 39
       3.8.9   The WHO Working Group on Sustainable Financing ... 40
3.9   Conclusions... 42
References... 43

4 **WHO Negotiations on a Pandemic Treaty and the International
   Health Regulations Adopted in 2024**......................... 47
   4.1   Introduction... 47
   4.2   A Binding International Treaty Within the WHO 48
   4.3   Treaty Negotiations: Progress, Tensions and Obstacles 49
   4.4   Country Positions: Interests, Tensions and Alliances 50
   4.5   The Failure of Negotiations on a Binding Treaty to Prevent
          Future Pandemics 51
   4.6   The New International Health Regulations.................. 53
   4.7   Reference to Financing 54
   4.8   Creation of a Committee of States Parties.................. 54
   4.9   "Progress" for the United States 55
   References... 55

5 **Building a Latin American and Caribbean Medicines Agency** 57
   5.1   Introduction... 57
   5.2   General Context....................................... 58
   5.3   The International Council for Harmonization of Technical
          Requirements for Pharmaceuticals for Human Use 59
   5.4   Suggested Principles and Goals for a Latin American Food
          and Drug Regulatory Agency 61
   5.5   Concluding Remarks................................... 62
   References... 62

**6   From the Concept of "Essential Medicines" to That of "Medical
      Countermeasures"** 63
      6.1   Introduction 63
      6.2   The Concept of Essential Medicines 63
      6.3   The Model List of Essential Medicines 64
      6.4   Action Programme on Essential Medicines 66
      6.5   Components of a National Pharmaceutical Policy 66
      6.6   Current Situation and Outlook 67
      6.7   Where Does the Expression "Medical Countermeasures"
             or "Health Countermeasures" Come From? 67
      References 68

**7   The Announcement of the United States' Withdrawal From
      the WHO: "Shooting Oneself in the Foot..."** 71
      7.1   Introduction 71
      7.2   US Presence in the WHO 71
      7.3   A Blow to the Multilateral System 72
      7.4   A False Justification, and a Reckless Decision for
             Global Health 73
      7.5   Conclusion 74
      References 75

8   Final Remarks and Possible Way Forward 77

Appendix: Recent South Centre Research Papers on Public Health 81

Index 87

About the Author

Germán Velásquez   is Special Adviser, Policy and Health of the South Centre in Geneva, Switzerland. Previously, he was Director of the Secretariat on Public Health, Innovation and Intellectual Property at WHO. He represented WHO at the WTO TRIPS Council from 2001 to 2010. He is the author and co-author of numerous publications on health economics and medicines, health insurance schemes, globalization, international trade agreements, intellectual property and access to medicines.

He obtained a Master's degree in Economics and a PhD in Health Economics from Sorbonne University, Paris. In 2010, he received a Honoris Causa PhD on Public Health from the University of Caldas, Colombia, and in 2015 he received another Honoris Causa PhD from the Faculty of Medicine of the Complutense University of Madrid, Spain.

Abbreviations and Acronyms

AMLAC	Medicines Agency for Latin America and the Caribbean
AMR	Antimicrobial resistance
BRICS	Brazil, Russia, India, China and South Africa
CELAC	Community of Latin American and Caribbean States
CEPI	Coalition for innovations in epidemic preparedness
COVAX	Financing facility for access to COVID-19 vaccines (COVAX Facility)
COVID-19	Coronavirus disease
EPI	Expanded Programme on Immunization
FIF	Financial Intermediary Funds
GAVI	the Global Alliance for Vaccines
GAVI COVAX AMC	GAVI COVAX Advance Market Commitment (AMC) for COVID-19 vaccines
GDP	Gross Domestic Product
GHAs	Global Health Actors (international players in the field of global health)
GMPs	Good manufacturing practices
GPA	Global Programme on AIDS
GSG	Global Steering Group for Impact Investment
ICDRA	International Conference of Drug Regulatory Authorities
ICH	The International Council for Harmonisation of Technical Requirements for Pharmaceuticals for Human Use
IHR	International Health Regulations (2005)
IMF	International Monetary Fund
INB	Intergovernmental negotiating body to draft and negotiate a WHO convention, agreement or other international instrument on pandemic prevention, preparedness and response
MPP	Medicines Patent Pool
MSF	Médecins Sans Frontières (Doctors Without Borders)
NAM	Non-Aligned Movement
NGO	Non-governmental organisation

ODA	Official development assistance
OECD	Organisation for Economic Co-operation and Development
PABS	Pathogen Access and Benefit Sharing System
PAHO	Pan American Health Organization
PDP	Product Development Partnership
PEPFAR	The U.S. President's Emergency Plan for AIDS Relief
PHEIC	Public health emergency of international concern
PPP	Public–private partnership
R&D	Research and Development
SDGs	Sustainable Development Goals
TDR	WHO Special Programme on Research and Training in Tropical Diseases
TRIPS	Agreement on Trade-Related Aspects of Intellectual Property Rights
UN	United Nations
UNAIDS	The Joint United Nations Programme on HIV/AIDS
UNCTAD	UN Trade and Development
UNDP	United Nations Development Programme
UNICEF	United Nations Children's Fund
WHA	World Health Assembly
WHO	World Health Organization
WIPO	World Intellectual Property Organization
WTO	World Trade Organization

Chapter 1
Introduction

Since the early 2000s, discussions, financing, declarations and resolutions on what might be described as global health have become increasingly dispersed. Alongside the World Health Organization (WHO), the specialized health agency of the United Nations system, there are now other organizations that deal with health issues and, in many cases, have much larger budgets than the WHO. These include the World Bank, the Global Fund to Fight AIDS, Tuberculosis and Malaria and the Gavi Alliance for Vaccines.

There is a proliferation of international players in the health sector today (Chap. 2). A certain "politically correct" discourse continues to insist that the WHO is the global coordinating body, but in practice, things seem to work rather differently. In reality, a substantial proportion of global public health financing is channelled through a number of other institutions and groups.

We are not in an era of change, but rather in a change of era. We have moved from the imperfect public multilateralism of healthcare to an era based on public–private management financed by a multiplicity of public and private players, including philanthropists.

The multiplicity and diversity of the objectives and interests of the new players in global health are probably positive aspects, but it's clear that, in the actions of the various players, there can be juxtapositions, inconsistencies and even contradictions.

Perhaps the most significant element of this new era is the fact that the G7 countries have decided that financing for global health must come from both private and public sources. "Mobilizing private funds in addition to public funds, including through sustainable financing, has become a matter of urgency" (G7, 2023).

The systematic involvement of the private sector in health financing and management is now being encouraged, raising serious concerns on how to guarantee equity and universal coverage, particularly in developing countries.

To date, the percentage of regular contributions to the World Health Organization's regular budget, i.e., the public contribution, represents just 16 percent of the WHO

© The Author(s), under exclusive license to Springer Nature
Switzerland AG 2025
G. Velásquez, *Negotiating Global Health Policies*, SpringerBriefs in Public
Health, https://doi.org/10.1007/978-3-031-99847-8_1

budget (WHO, 2022). The good news is that the 75th World Health Assembly (WHA—the decision-making body of the WHO) in 2022 approved an increase in regular State contributions from member countries to reach a level of 50 percent of the 2022–2023 core budget by the 2030–2031 biennium (WHO, 2022). However, even if WHO member countries were to comply with this increase, the total increase in contributions to the organization's regular budget would only represent an increase of US$1.2 billion, which could be compared with some perplexity to the billions that will or aspire to be managed by entities and mechanisms outside the WHO.

In addition, the COVID pandemic revealed serious flaws in the response to a major health crisis. In an attempt to remedy this, and recognizing that future pandemics are inevitable, the WHA decided to prepare a Treaty to respond to future pandemics. One of the central issues for the WHA in May/June 2024 was the discussion, or rather negotiation, of this Treaty (Chap. 3). Discussions around this treaty have been tense and have so far been inconclusive. To ensure that the errors and injustices committed during COVID-19 can be effectively remedied, negotiations should be conducted with greater ambition, particularly with a view to establishing a binding international treaty.

To make progress towards achieving this goal, the revision of the Intergovernmental negotiating body to draft and negotiate a WHO convention, agreement or other international instrument on pandemic prevention, preparedness and response (INB), and of the International Health Regulations (Chap. 4) must go hand in hand. These two parallel processes on very similar issues often led to overlap and even confusion, for example, over which document discussed which issues. Several observers saw these parallel negotiations as a tactic by industrialized countries to avoid the inclusion of certain elements defended by developing countries. The urgency with which the United States and the European Union approved the IHR at WHA 2024, while leaving negotiations on a pandemic treaty open, was undoubtedly due to the industrialized countries' wish that negotiations on the pandemic treaty should not "contaminate" the IHR on issues such as access to vaccines, medicines and diagnostic tools.

The two and a half years of negotiations around the Intergovernmental Negotiating Body (INB), with relatively little progress compared to the challenges that a new pandemic could pose to the world, and the mediocre results of the IHR 2024 revision confirm the impasse in which the multilateral system finds itself.

If the leadership of the so-called global health system became concentrated in the hands of the G7 countries, this would lead to an impasse in the multilateral public health system. In the light of the obstacles that could arise at multilateral level in the adoption of global solutions, regional initiatives and solutions could provide a response (Chap. 5). Negotiations in the context of the Intergovernmental Negotiating Body (INB) at the WHO have emphasized the need for regional solutions.

This could include the regional manufacture of vaccines and medical supplies, the creation of regional medicines agencies with sanitary standards that promote regional health and production (the Latin American and Caribbean Medicines Agency—AMLAC), proposed by some Latin American countries, or the African

Medicines Agency, currently being created), as well as a regional approach to intellectual property standards, using the flexibilities of the Agreement on Trade-Related Aspects of Intellectual Property Rights (TRIPS).

The book continues with a discussion of a central concept in global health, that of essential medicines (Chap. 6). This is a striking example of how international negotiations can weaken and distort the basic concepts of public health developed by the WHO and many WHO member countries over decades. We refer to the manner in which the concept of "essential medicines" is currently being replaced with the concept of "medical countermeasures", thus stripping the former concept of its radically innovative nature and its capacity to promote social justice in health systems.

The World Health Organization is an example of the weakening of the multilateral system. By addressing the various issues raised here—the different stakeholders, the financing, the treaties, the basic concepts—we attempt to show how endangered the organization is. This might inspire those who are concerned about the best way to safeguard a healthy life for all.

Finally, the book concludes with a discussion on the announcement of the United States' withdrawal from the WHO.

This book presents the reflections and research carried out by the author at the South Centre to provide policymakers, researchers and other stakeholders with information and analysis on issues relating to public health, access to medicines and ongoing international negotiations to prepare for and prevent future pandemics.

References

G7. (2023). Impact investment initiative for global health. G7 Hiroshima Summit. https://www.mofa.go.jp/files/100507018.pdf.

WHO. (2022). Report of the meeting of the working group on sustainable financing. Doc. EB/WGSF/7/4, 9 May 2022.

Chapter 2
Current Challenges and Possible Future Scenarios for Global Health

2.1 Introduction

To think about possible future scenarios for global health, it is important to look at the past and try to understand the present. In the 1980s, the main global players in health were the WHO, the United Nations Children's Fund (UNICEF) and (through bilateral cooperation) the United States of America and Northern European countries, particularly the Netherlands, Denmark, Sweden and Norway, as well as some non-profit NGOs such as Médecins Sans Frontières (MSF) and Medicus Mundi.

Today, we are witnessing a proliferation of international players in the field of global health (GHAs—Global Health Actors): WHO, UNICEF, UNAIDS, Unitaid, UNCTAD, WTO, WIPO, UNDP, FAO, the United Nations Secretariat in New York,[1] the International Monetary Fund (IMF), the World Bank,[2] and the regional development banks, the G7 and G20, the G77+ China, the Non-Aligned Movement (NAM), BRICS, The Global Fund, public–private partnerships such as the GAVI Alliance or COVAX, CEPI, the pharmaceutical industry, certain private companies with the so-called "social responsibility" projects, philanthropic foundations such as Bill & Melinda Gates, George Soros and others. Melinda Gates, George Soros or Bloomberg, professional associations from different health disciplines, non-profit and for-profit non-governmental organizations, universities and even large private consultancy groups such as McKinsey or Accenture.

We are not in an era of change, but rather in a change of era. We are moving from imperfect public multilateralism in healthcare to an era based on public–private

---

[1] For several years, high-level panels or political meetings have been organised at UN level on health-related issues, for example on AIDS/HIV, tuberculosis and the recent high-level meeting on pandemic prevention, preparedness and response (20 September 2023).

[2] Including the new Pandemic Fund.

© The Author(s), under exclusive license to Springer Nature Switzerland AG 2025
G. Velásquez, *Negotiating Global Health Policies*, SpringerBriefs in Public Health, https://doi.org/10.1007/978-3-031-99847-8_2

management financed by a multiplicity of public and private players, including philanthropists.

For the past 3 years, WHO member countries have been negotiating the reform of the 2005 International Health Regulations (IHR) and working on the drafting of a potentially binding international instrument negotiated by the Intergovernmental Negotiating Body (INB) to prevent and prepare the world for future pandemics such as COVID-19. The implementation of these instruments, if something concrete and effective were to be achieved, would be in the hands of the WHO, one of the many players in global health.

All these bodies, mechanisms and groups—the list is not exhaustive—have different dynamics, objectives, priorities, financial resources, working methods, action strategies and interests. Not all have public interest as a priority, and among those that do, not all pursue or promote it in the same manner. Some current narratives insist that all these actors should be coordinated by the WHO, but in reality much of the funding for global public health is channelled to many other institutions or groups, and although the narrative insists that the WHO coordinates, it does not have, or use, the instruments available to govern global public health. Moreover, there are already discordant voices within this discourse, such as those who suggest that the United Nations Secretariat in New York (Moon & Kickbusch, 2021) should be the coordinator, or those who argue—like former New Zealand Prime Minister Helen Clark—for the creation of a high-level panel of experts ("a body independent of the WHO") to "oversee the WHO and other actors" (Clark, 2023).

The multiplicity and diversity of the objectives and interests of the new players in global health is probably a positive aspect, but it is clear that the situation is complex, sometimes confusing and, as we are beginning to see today from the actions of the various players, there can be juxtapositions, inconsistencies or contradictions. In this respect, it has been observed that "the renewed focus on health systems is welcome, but many global health actors are simply putting old wine in new bottles. They claim that their selective practices help to strengthen systems, when in fact the opposite is true" (Marchal et al., 2009).

Of all the above players, perhaps the most powerful is the G7, the group of the world's richest countries (Canada, France, Germany, Italy, Japan, the United Kingdom and the United States), which describes itself as representing the leading industrialized nations. Its members want to be recognized for their commitment to democracy, the rule of law, economic prosperity and working together to solve global problems (Kickbusch et al., 2022). They are the "ricchi e buoni" (as Nicoletta Dentico would say) (Dentico, 2020).

This chapter analyses the new multiple players in healthcare (public and private, including philanthropic) and, on this basis, attempts to sketch out possible scenarios for the future.

In this new era dominated by a diversity of World Health Assemblies (WHAs), powerful new players could and are already influencing the direction of global health by proposing different possible scenarios that do not clearly prioritize access to the resources needed to guarantee public health.

Although the financial resources available for public health have now increased, its management has become more complex, and its objectives do not always follow clear interests that are consistent with health as a right and not as a commodity. While the public sector aims to achieve the common good, private sector intervention cannot be dissociated from more or less apparent commercial interests (Velásquez, 2023).

In the 1980s, global health funding was multilateral and public; today, it depends on ad hoc contributions from governments and the private and philanthropic sector (e.g. GAVI Alliance, CEPI, COVAX, World Bank, Bill & Melinda Gates, Bloomberg). The guidelines for the use of these funds are largely imposed by the G7 and G20, which, since the COVID-19 pandemic, have taken an increasing interest in the direction of action in the health sector.

The differences between the objectives, dynamics, methodologies, etc. of the GHAs are making it increasingly difficult to manage global health despite the insistence on the WHO leading role, mainly, as has been said, because most of the funds go to entities or mechanisms over which the WHO has no decision-making power (Velásquez, 2023).

2.2   The World Bank and the International Monetary Fund

As Prah Ruger points out, although the World Bank was set up in 1946 to finance the reconstruction of Europe after the Second World War, it has not yet been fully operational:

> The Bank is now a considerable force in the health, nutrition and population (HNP) sector in developing countries. In fact, from having virtually no presence in global health, the Bank has become the world's largest financier of health-related projects, currently committing more than $1 billion a year (2005) to new health, nutrition and population projects. It is also one of the main supporters of the fight against HIV/AIDS, with commitments of over 1.6 billion dollars in recent years.

> The World Bank has announced a $14 billion rapid response package and plans to deploy up to $160 billion over the next 15 months. Instead of using its Health, Nutrition and Population Division, which has expertise in health, most of this aid ($8 billion) will be channelled through the International Finance Corporation, the Bank's private sector financing arm. This structure was chosen despite its lack of experience in setting up public health systems and the accumulated evidence of the mediocre (and costly) results of public-private partnerships in the health sector (Prah Ruger, 2011).

The President of the World Bank, David Malpass, made it clear during the COVID-19 pandemic that his institution's support was conditional on structural adjustment policies imposing deregulation (for example, encouraging private markets in the healthcare sector) or trade liberalization (Malpass, 2020).

The IMF's main response to the COVID-19 crisis was, as it had done before the pandemic, to encourage the countries affected by the crisis to apply for conventional loans, (...). It was noted that:

These loans are subject to controversial conditionalities: reforms that must be introduced before the money is disbursed. These conditionalities have negative effects on the health of the population because they include ill-conceived policy measures, such as budget cuts, reducing the number and salaries of health and social workers, weakening labour protection or encouraging privatisation (Kentikelenis et al., 2020).

The question remains: to what extent is it acceptable for a country to borrow to finance its current healthcare expenditure? Accepting loans from the World Bank (or IMF) forces countries to make additional debt repayments, which may make it more difficult to finance health systems. In other words, during the pandemic, the IMF and World Bank pursued policies that gave priority to conventional financing solutions, which could have negative consequences for health outcomes.

Is there an alternative, ask the authors of The Lancet article entitled "Softening the blow of the pandemic: will the International Monetary Fund and World Bank make things worse"? (Kentikelenis et al., 2020). We agree that there is. Here are some of the relevant points made by the authors:

– investing in public health with universal coverage. Public health systems, which serve the most vulnerable, need adequate funding to recruit and retain health and social workers, manage facilities and purchase equipment and medicines. These investments would help to guarantee universal coverage.
– avoid the conditions that generally accompany these loans
– announce an immediate debt moratorium with public and private creditors, such as that implemented in certain high-income countries, in order to channel funds to deal with the pandemic.
– The authors warn that "for decades, international financial institutions have pursued policies that have undermined public health systems, allowing billions of people to continue to be deprived of adequate healthcare. The COVID-19 pandemic is an opportunity to do things differently" (Kentikelenis et al., 2020).

2.2.1 World Bank Intermediate Prevention, Preparedness and Response Fund

The new Financial Intermediary Fund (FIF) for pandemic prevention, preparedness and response "will provide a dedicated stream of additional, long-term financing to strengthen pandemic prevention, preparedness, and response (PPR) capabilities in low- and middle-income countries" (World Bank, 2022). The World Bank is the administrator of the FIF and hosts the Secretariat. Since the launch of the FIF by the World Bank and WHO on 30 June 2022, the initiative has been the subject of much writing, comment and speculation. Some media had anticipated a fund of 50 billion dollars. However, this figure no longer appears in the Bank's factual information (United Nations News, 2021).

2.2.2   Goals and Roles of the World Bank FIF

The World Bank's Board of Directors authorized the establishment of this new fund on 30 June 2022, with the backing of G20 members. It was formally introduced at a high-level gathering held on the sides of the joint G20 finance and health ministers' meeting in Bali on 11 November 2022 (The Pandemic Fund, 2025).

In addition to representatives from foundations and civil society organizations, the FIF Board has equal representation of sovereign donors and the governments of nations that are likely to carry out the programme (co-investors). The WHO will offer technical assistance and take part as a non-voting observer, while the World Bank will administer the Fund.

Australia, Canada, China, the European Commission, France, Germany, India, Indonesia, Italy, Japan, the Netherlands, New Zealand, Norway, the Republic of Korea, Saudi Arabia, Singapore, South Africa, Spain, Switzerland, the United Arab Emirates, the United States, the Bill and Melinda Gates Foundation, the Rockefeller Foundation and the Wellcome Trust have all committed more than $1.6 billion, according to the Financial Intermediary Fund.

Funding from the Fund is available for "One Health" initiatives that acknowledge the interdependence of human and animal health and how it is related to the health of the ecosystems they share. The Fund also receives business sector contributions and can be used to fund antimicrobial resistance (AMR) related activities.

2.2.3   Comments and Reactions to World Bank Reports on the FIF

Emily Bass and Asia Russell, the two authors previously mentioned, issued their initial remarks about the new fund in July 2022, 1 month after the FIF's creation was announced: "This fund, enthusiastically supported by the United States, is, in its current form, doomed to failure". Numerous organizations have pointed out potentially fatal flaws in the project, including a problematic governance approach, a small list of implementing entities, and the lack of a true strategy to ensure equity, access and impact. These groups include the World Health Organization's Council on Health Economics for All, the Centers for Disease Control and Prevention in Africa, and a variety of seasoned activist groups and coalitions. The Financial Intermediary Fund (FIF) for Pandemic Prevention, Preparedness and Response, the newest global health fund, now seems destined to fail (Bass & Russell, 2022a).

Bass and Russell in their paper "Back from the brink" once more voiced their grave concerns and reservations in "Think Global Health" regarding the role of the US government and World Bank management in the establishment and direction of the Pandemic Fund during the second meeting of the World Bank's governors in October 2022, which was chaired by David Malpass, the bank's director (Bass & Russell, 2022b).

Many civil society organizations question the efficacy of the new fund if private actors are primarily in charge of its implementation. For example, Marco Angelo of the Belgian civil society organization Wemos stated that "development actors should prioritise public provision over private provision, particularly in the case of primary health care, as the Lancet Commission on Primary Health Care recently emphasised". He said, "Private provision negatively affects equitable access when it is not integrated into the public health financing system; when it is integrated, on the other hand, it can present many challenges" (Bretton Woods Project, 2022).

In response to the World Bank's FIF proposal, 33 civil society organizations signed a joint letter stating: "The World Bank and the World Health Organization (WHO) have estimated that $10.5 billion of external financing will be needed over the next five years for investments at country, regional, and global levels to build capacity in low- and middle-income countries" (WEMOS, Eurodad, 2022). In order to make the FIF proposal truly inclusive, the 33 organizations insist on a global public investment approach and offer a number of recommendations on governance, finance and private sector engagement. One of the top priorities should be to strengthen the public sector. A robust public health system is the most crucial instrument for guaranteeing an efficient and fair response to health catastrophes, including pandemics, as the COVID-19 pandemic has made abundantly evident (WEMOS, Eurodad, 2022).

Similarly, Helen Clark, co-chair of the Independent Panel on Pandemic Preparedness and Response, emphasized at the September 2023 UN General Assembly that "a global public investment model is needed to pool funds to support low- and middle-income countries" (Clark, 2023).

The World Bank states that "USD 350 million was the amount of the allocation that was approved by the Board". Since the Board intended for this initial request for proposals to be a learning exercise, the allocation was very limited in relation to the Pandemic Fund's overall resources. Taking into consideration the lessons acquired for the benefit of future applicants, the Pandemic Fund said in early 2023 that it would issue another call for ideas (World Bank, 2023).

Any funding for pandemic preparedness, prevention and response must follow a human rights-based approach.

One of the top priorities must be to strengthen the public sector. A robust public health system is the most crucial instrument for guaranteeing an efficient and fair response to health emergencies, including pandemics, as the COVID-19 pandemic has made abundantly evident (World Bank, 2023). Despite its lofty objective, the FIF has only secured US$1.6 billion in promises from the aforementioned contributors by the end of 2022.

2.3   G7 - G20 - BRICS

The Group of Seven (G7) is a group of heads of state and government created at the initiative of the United States of America during the first oil crisis of the 1970s. Initially, the G7 comprised just five countries (the United States, Germany, France, the United Kingdom and Japan). But Italy and Canada soon joined the group. Russia was included in 1997 to form the G8, but was excluded in March 2014 following the annexation of Crimea (ECONOMIQUEMENT.FR, 2025).

The Group of Seven (G7) and the Group of Twenty (G20) are informal governance clubs that hold annual summits of heads of state to discuss issues of global importance. The G7 is a more homogenous and intimate group, which has been meeting for decades. It is a sub-group—a club within a club—of the newer and more diverse G20, which represents the emerging multipolar world order (Heinrich-Böll-Stiftung, 2016).

Before the G7 began to take an interest in global health, it was noted that the WHO Secretariat was heavily influenced by "representatives of the governments of the United States, the European Union, Switzerland, Canada, Japan and Australia, who preferred a weak organisation that would serve, or at least not interfere with, the financial and commercial interests of their food and pharmaceutical industries" (Velásquez, 2016). The countries mentioned above practically coincide with the members of the G7. The relationship (if any) between the WHO and the G7 is not clear, but it can be assumed that G7 members do not adopt decisions, strategies or policies in multilateral bodies such as the WHO that run counter to what they have agreed within the G7. For example, during the COVID-19 crisis, the G7 as a group announced its support for the purchase of vaccines: "COVAX welcomes the G7 commitments to provide an additional 870 million doses to support equitable access to vaccines in 2021 and 2022, as well as the target to provide at least half of these doses by 2021" (WHO, 2021).

The world is facing multiple crises affecting global health, such as climate change, wars and armed conflicts, and recent pandemics such as COVID-19. Against this backdrop, the Group of Seven (G7) in Hiroshima and the G7 Health Ministers' meeting in Nagasaki (Japan) in May 2023 drew up a global health agenda for the seven industrialized countries (G7, 2023).

In recent years, the financial burden of healthcare has increased worldwide, particularly in low- and middle-income countries. In this context, the G7 communiqué states, "*it has become urgent to mobilise private and public funds, including through sustainable financing*" (G7, 2023).[3]

In early 2023, the G7 announced the intention to launch the Triple I for Global Health (Impact Investment Initiative for Global Health) in the margins of the United Nations General Assembly High Level Meetings in September 2023. On that date, a political declaration of the high-level meeting on universal health coverage

---

[3] Emphasis by the author.

"Universal health coverage: Expanding our ambition for health and well-being in a post-COVID world" was adopted in New York (United Nations, 2023).

In point 36, the declaration recognizes that the financing of health systems poses significant problems in low- and middle-income countries, where more than a third of national health expenditure is out-of-pocket and where public expenditure accounts for less than 40 percent of primary health care funding; international aid funding accounts for only 0.2 percent of global health expenditure but can represent a significant percentage of national health expenditure, reaching around 30 percent in low-income countries (UNGA, 2023).

Further on, point 73 of the declaration states:

> Explore, encourage and promote a range of innovative incentives and funding mechanisms for health research and development, including *a stronger and more transparent public-private partnership*[4] (...) recognising the important role of the private sector in the research and development of innovative medicines (UNGA, 2023, Point 76).

The G7 Japan Communiqué (2023) envisaged as a next step inviting development finance institutions, public development banks, multilateral development banks, private companies and other relevant organizations to consider joining in the co-creation of such an initiative to support and develop a framework for mobilizing private sector investment. A Secretariat would raise awareness, collect data, disseminate good practice, convene working groups and organize forums. The Secretariat would collaborate with implementation/knowledge partners, including the Global Steering Group for Impact Investment (GSG), the Impact Taskforce and the Bill & Melinda Gates Foundation (G7, 2023).

Further on, point 105 of the declaration states:

> Call upon the relevant entities of the United Nations development system, within their respective mandates, recognizing the key role of the World Health Organization as the directing and coordinating authority for international health activities, in accordance with its Constitution, and of the United Nations country teams, under the leadership of the revitalized resident coordinators, within their respective mandates, *as well as other global development and health actors, including civil society, the private sector* and academia, to assist and support countries in their efforts to achieve universal health coverage at country level, in accordance with their respective national contexts, priorities and expertise. (UNGA 2023, Point 105).

The G20 was created in 1999 on the initiative of the finance ministers and central bank governors of the G7 countries, with the aim of including emerging countries in discussions on the global economy. In addition to the G7 countries, the G20 includes Argentina, Australia, Brazil, China, India, Indonesia, Mexico, Saudi Arabia, South Africa, South Korea and Turkey, as well as representatives of the European Union. The G20 countries account for almost all of global gross domestic product (GDP), of world trade and two-thirds of the world's population (Government of Spain, 2025). The African Union recently joined the group.

---

[4] Emphasis by the author.

The G20, which met for the first time in Washington in November 2008, is now the main international forum for cooperation and consultation on economic and financial issues. As such, official institutions such as the IMF and the World Bank are invited to G20 meetings (ECONOMIQUEMENT.FR, 2025). In 2017, G20 health ministers met for the first time to discuss global health and issued a communiqué outlining their health priorities, as the G7 has done for years. As these political clubs carry considerable political and economic weight, their respective global health agendas can influence both global health priorities and those of other countries and actors (McBride et al., 2019).

Another smaller club—which includes some G20 members—is the BRICS, an alliance of emerging economies: Brazil, Russia, India, China and South Africa. In August 2023, at the 15th anniversary of the BRICS, South African President Cyril Ramaphosa announced that Saudi Arabia, Argentina, Egypt, the United Arab Emirates, Ethiopia and Iran had been invited to join the bloc from 1 January 2024 (Liberation.fr, 2023).

In 2001, Jim O'Neill, an economist at the investment bank Goldman Sachs, coined the acronym "BRIC" for Brazil, Russia, India and China. These were large middle-income countries with rapidly growing economies. He predicted that they could become the world's leading economies by 2050. In 2006, the four countries decided to join forces to form the group. South Africa joined the group in 2010 (BBC NEWS Afrique, 2023). For many, this group represents the prospect of a unified geopolitical bloc which, among other objectives, can help to reframe the development of global health within a new set of ideas and values.

In July 2011, health ministers from Brazil, Russia, India, China and South Africa met in Beijing for the first BRICS Health Ministers' Meeting. In what subsequently became known as the "Beijing Declaration", the ministers pledged to initiate, advocate and support a series of global health measures (BRICS Information Centre, 2011).

In addition, the health ministers agreed to "promote the BRICS as a forum for coordination, cooperation and consultation on relevant global public health issues" (BRICS Information Centre, 2011). On 22 May 2012, they met again in Geneva to discuss cooperation on health for their citizens "as well as for the whole world" (BRICS Information Centre, 2012).

Harmer et al. reviewed more than 800 articles on the subject in order to determine the possible influence of the BRICS on global health and, if so, how this influence has been conceptualized and recorded in the literature (Harmer et al., 2013).

The first positive aspect of Harmer's study is that the BRICS health alliance could lead to concrete collective action in favour of global health at some undetermined point in the future and, above all, that this group has the potential to reshape Western models of global health governance and development aid.

On the other hand, a more pessimistic reading of the literature reviewed highlights that the BRICS have so far been unable to cooperate or coordinate their actions or influence on specific global health issues (for example, reform of the WHO or universal health coverage).

Harmer's study found little evidence that the BRICS are influencing global health, although some BRICS countries are becoming more vocal and active in shaping and even leading global health movements, such as universal healthcare coverage or the production of generic medicines. The study notes that:

> The various summits and meetings of BRICS health ministers suggest that there is political will for collective action and that political leaders now recognise that their health ministers have the opportunity to steer the global health agenda in a new direction. The challenge is to build on this momentum and turn political will into action (Harmer et al., 2013).

The above analysis of the three groups of countries (G7, G20, BRICS) raises a number of questions:

- How do their priorities fit in with the mandates and negotiations underway at the WHO, the multilateral body to which the G7, G20 and BRICS countries belong?
- Will the WHO provide a group of countries with specific technical and/or financial assistance on health issues?
- What's the need or benefit for regional groups, or groups of friendly countries, to define health programmes to which they have already subscribed as members of the multilateral organization, the WHO?
- How can we ensure that the issues defined as health priorities for the G7, G20 and BRICS countries are consistent with the commitments made by these countries to the WHO?
- Who will support and help countries that do not belong to any of these groups?

2.4   The Group of 77 and China

The Declaration of the Group of 77 and China (G77 + China) of September 2023 in Havana, Cuba, states in its point 6: "We stress the urgent need for a comprehensive reform of the international financial architecture and a more inclusive and coordinated approach to global financial governance, with greater emphasis on cooperation among countries, including through increasing the representation of developing countries in global decision and policy-making bodies which will contribute to enhance the capacities of developing countries to access and develop science, technology and innovation".

G77 + China, which now has 134 countries represented at the Havana summit, is calling for "greater representation of developing countries in global decision-making and policy-making bodies". This call refers to the G7, which has seven countries, the G20, which has 20, and the BRICS, which has five or eleven (the six countries recently invited). If decisions are taken by the G7, the G20 or the BRICS, more than 100 countries will be excluded from decision-making.

The G77+ China statement continues in point 29: "We call upon the international community and relevant bodies of the United Nations system to take urgent action to promote unhindered, timely and equitable access for developing countries to health-related measures, products and technologies necessary to deal with the current and future pandemic prevention preparedness and responses. These include through financing, health systems strengthening, building capacity, ensuring sustainability of supply chains, technology transfer and know-how for local and regional manufacturing and production of medical countermeasures, including medicines, vaccines, therapeutics, diagnostics, health technologies and other health products in developing countries".

This appeal is addressed "to the relevant bodies of the United Nations system", i.e., the multilateral system.

2.5 The Non-Aligned Movement

The Non-Aligned Movement (NAM) was created during the Cold War as an organization of States that did not want to align themselves with either the United States of America or the Soviet Union but sought to remain neutral in the confrontation between the great powers of the time. The basic concept of the group was born in 1955 during discussions at the Asia-Africa conference in Bandung, Indonesia.

As Li, Uribe and Danish pointed out in a study by the South Centre:

> The non-aligned movement was born out of the need felt by the new post-colonial nations not to be forced into a political or military bloc during the Cold War. Now that the international community is once again faced with growing geopolitical tensions, the principles of non-alignment have resurfaced in the South, giving the Non-Aligned Movement the opportunity to become a major force in shaping a new international order (Li et al., 2023).

The Movement's first summit conference was held in Belgrade, Yugoslavia, in September 1961. The Movement currently has 120 members: 53 from Africa, 39 from Asia, 26 from Latin America and the Caribbean and 2 from Europe (Belarus and Azerbaijan) (Drishti The Vision, 2019).

Since the early 1990s, the health ministers of the Non-Aligned Movement have met on the first or second day of the World Health Assembly (WHA). The Director-General of the WHO attended the deliberations, but because of the wide diversity of countries that make up the Movement, the statements were rather general, and, in the end, few concrete declarations were made on the various issues that would be discussed at the World Health Assembly in the following days.

However, during the COVID-19 pandemic, the health ministers of the Non-Aligned Movement sent a strong and clear message of support to the WHO in defence of multilateralism in the field of health:

> ... the member countries agreed on the importance of solidarity and international cooperation to guarantee global access to medicines, vaccines and medical equipment, and to prevent the negative effects of the pandemic on the economy (Permana, 2020).

> More than six decades after its creation, the Non-Aligned Movement stands at a crucial juncture, where the consolidation of non-alignment among developing countries can help foster solidarity, promote collaboration and defend the interests of developing countries in the reconfiguration of global governance. Meeting these challenges requires unprecedented levels of international cooperation, both North-South and South-South. As a grouping of

non-aligned countries, the Non-Aligned Movement could play an important role in the fight against global fragmentation, the promotion of solidarity and the strengthening of multilateralism (Li et al., 2023).

In this context, the role of the Non-Aligned Movement should be to influence the debates within the WHO governing bodies (World Health Assembly and Executive Board) by proposing and defending the interests of developing countries in critical areas such as access to pharmaceutical products and medical technologies, the promotion of local production and universal health coverage.

2.6   Philanthropy's Foray into Global Health

The history of modern philanthropy can be traced back to the late nineteenth and early twentieth centuries, with Andrew Carnegie and the steel empire in Pittsburgh and John Rockefeller and the "black gold" of oil in California (Dentico, 2020). As Rob Reich writes, "growing inequality will be the enemy of civil coexistence and certainly the friend of philanthropy" (Reich et al., 2016). Neither Carnegie nor Rockefeller (or a modern-day Bill Gates) ever questioned the goal of unlimited wealth. Carnegie did not hesitate to write at the end of the 1990s that inequality was inevitable and that it was the price of progress:

> The contrast between the palace of the millionaire and the small house of the worker that we see in our time only serves to give the measure of the change that is taking place in our civilisation. This change is by no means deplorable; it should be welcomed as a great advantage (...) (Kolbert, 2018).

The world of philanthropy raises ethical questions about unbridled enrichment and the social inequalities to which it contributes. With regard to current healthcare philanthropy, it is important to examine where the fortunes behind it come from and where the respective funds are invested. For example, the Ford, Rockefeller, W.K. Kellogg and Robert Wood Johnson foundations (as well as the Bill and Melinda Gates Foundation) have generated resources by investing in pharmaceutical and food companies, among others (Stuckler et al., 2011).

David McCoy et al. analysed 1094 grants awarded between January 1998 and December 2007 by the Bill & Melinda Gates Foundation and found that the total value of these grants was $8.95 billion, of which $5.82 billion was distributed to just 20 organizations, including organizations with a role in global public health such as the WHO, GAVI Alliance, the World Bank and the Global Fund to Fight AIDS, Tuberculosis and Malaria (McCoy et al., 2009).

These sums represent significant percentages of the budgets of the beneficiary entities; for example, in the case of the WHO, the Bill & Melinda Gates Foundation is the second largest non-state contributor to the organization's budget.

An analysis of philanthropic organizations' funds devoted to health suggests the need to address a number of problem areas:

– Where do these funds come from?

- To what extent do these contributions change the priorities of beneficiaries when donors identify issues for funding?
- What are the conditions required by foundations, such as participation in expert committees and/or in the beneficiaries' management bodies?
- What mechanisms are in place to avoid potential conflicts of interest?

2.7 Public–Private Partnerships in Global Healthcare

Public–private partnerships (PPPs) in healthcare were launched on the premise that they would create a win–win situation. However, Gro Harlem Brundtland, Director of the WHO (1998–2003), at her second round table with the International Federation of Pharmaceutical Manufacturers & Associations (IFPMA), said: "I recognise that the differences in objectives and responsibilities between the research-based pharmaceutical industry and the WHO make collaboration difficult".

This assumption of a "win–win" situation has contributed to the rapid increase in the number of PPPs in healthcare without clear evaluation mechanisms. If everyone wins, there shouldn't be too much danger, but if there are "winners" and "losers" in these partnerships, it's important to assess who wins and who loses.

According to Richter, PPPs involve certain "trade-offs" which make it necessary to examine the risks in terms of public policy and public interests (Richter, 2004). These risks are as follows:

- Commercial actors who use interaction with UN agencies to obtain political and commercial information in order to gain political influence and/or competitive advantage.
- Business players who use interaction to set the global public agenda in line with business interests.
- PPPs are far from being a new model for solving the problem of access to healthcare, particularly in developing countries. It is more an experiment than a "model".
- In the health sector, PPPs, as stated by Richter, back in 2004 in the aforementioned document, threaten the democratic and multilateral functioning on which the United Nations system and its specialized agencies, such as the WHO, are based (Richter, 2004). PPPs raise a number of concerns:

- Most of the products developed to date are incremental innovations.
- Its capacity is fairly modest.
- In some cases, they are in competition with each other. This can lead to overlap and wasted resources.
- Potential conflict of interest, as the private sector sits on public sector boards and advisory committees.
- In most PPPs for the development of pharmaceutical products, it is not known how intellectual property will be handled.

- In some cases, intermediate steps for non-neglected diseases (i.e., all other diseases that are not on the WHO list of "neglected diseases") are patented for commercial purposes, such as Product Development Partnership (PDP) adjuvants for malaria vaccines.
- PPPs are generally launched by donors from the North who decide on the problems and priorities of the South.

Torchia et al. (2015) carried out a systematic review of 46 articles published in international journals over the period 1990–2011. Six areas of PPP research were identified: effectiveness, benefits, public interest, country overview, efficiency and partners. The main findings suggest that, although PPPs are being used to address emerging public health problems internationally, questions about their effectiveness, efficiency and relevance remain unanswered.

In 2023, after the COVID-19 crisis, the first thing one might point out is that there are no internationally agreed fixed rules for the operation/behaviour of global public/private health partnerships such as GAVI or COVAX. If there were, we might ask who sets the rules and how they are applied. Generally speaking, in a neoliberal model, States have less and less influence over large private companies, many of which are now "transnationals" (Babacan, 2020), which have more and more power to limit or challenge the regulatory role of States (Hernández Zubizarreta, 2009).

The "ACT Accelerator" and COVAX were imposed as "the only global solution" for equitable access to vaccines, based on the public–private partnership model that has come to dominate global health management, propelled to a higher level by the COVID-19 crisis. This project was an experimental form of what might be called a "super or macro- public–private partnership", like the one that seems to be proposed nowadays by the G7, and the World Bank's Pandemic Fund (FIF) mentioned above.

The structural complexity of a super-public–private partnership masks the huge differences between the constituent partners when it comes to developed countries and their industry, giving pharmaceutical companies considerable power and making the public interest, transparency and accountability difficult to achieve.

The failure of COVAX would be grounds to question the legitimacy of the "macro-PPP" model in the field of global health; it raises the need to look for new avenues or solutions. (Tagmatarchi Storeng et al., 2021).

2.8 New Concepts: Health Security, Universal Health Coverage

Added to this already complex scenario is the new concept of "global health security" introduced by the G7 members. Not everyone is talking about the same thing when it comes to "health security" or "universal health coverage".

The concept of "health security" is increasingly referred to. The problem is that "there are various and incompatible definitions, incomplete elaboration of the concept of health security in public health operational terms, and insufficient reconciliation of the health security concept with community-based primary health care. More important, there are major differences in understanding and use of the concept in different settings. Policymakers in industrialized countries emphasize protection of their populations especially against external threats, for example terrorism and pandemics; while health workers and policymakers in developing countries and within the United Nations system understand the term in a broader public health context" (Aldis, 2008).

Within the WHO itself, the concept is used ambiguously as "global health security". Divergent interpretations, between developed and developing countries, are leading to uncertainty in the interpretation of the International Health Regulations (2005). "Some developing countries are beginning to doubt that internationally shared health surveillance data is used in their best interests" (Aldis, 2008).

As mentioned by W. Aldis, there is significant and growing opposition to the use of a "security" justification for global health cooperation, particularly from some developing countries, which is being ignored by representatives of the industrialized countries.

The problem with this conceptual difference is that, while the G7 clearly advocates the inclusion of the private sector as a structural player in global health, the resulting security is essentially that for a select few—the citizens of the countries of the North—rather than security for all.

Similarly, the gradual disappearance of the concept of essential medicines being replaced by that of "health security" (see Chap. 6) is problematic. This concept of "safety", applied here to healthcare, also raises many other questions.

2.9 The Role of Sustainable Development Objectives

The WHO thirteenth programme of work (2018–2023) states: "WHO will only succeed, however, if it bases its work on the Sustainable Development Goals (SDGs). The 2030 Agenda for Sustainable Development views health as vital for the future of our world. With a commitment to achieve Goal 3, which calls on all stakeholders to 'Ensure healthy lives and promote well-being for all at all ages'" (WHO, 2019).

Such references are also found in the G7 statements: "The COVID-19 pandemic (...) and the disruption of routine health services have moved us further away from achieving universal health coverage, the Millennium Development Goals and the Sustainable Development Goals (SDGs), in particular SDG 3 on health and well-being" (G7, 2022).

The Third Conference on Financing for Development (Addis Ababa, 13–16 July 2015), which was to identify the funds needed to implement the SDGs to be approved in July 2015 by the Heads of State attending the conference (United Nations, 2015), failed for lack of consensus (TWN, 2015). As the summit of Heads of State to adopt the SDGs was due to take place a few days later, the decision was taken to go ahead. In other words, the SDGs were announced without a consensus on their financing.

It was noted in this regard that "the Third International Conference on Financing for Development in Addis Ababa ended on 16 July in a climate of disagreement, with developed countries rejecting the creation of a global tax body and rejecting a compromise proposal by developing countries to strengthen the existing UN Committee of Tax Experts. Normally, when major conferences end in conflict and result in intergovernmental negotiations, there is a sense of exhilaration. This was not the case in Addis Ababa. On the contrary, developing countries and many United Nations officials were deeply disappointed, and civil society groups that had been following the free trade process for a year were outraged".[5]

It would not be wrong to say that the SDGs, to which all the international organizations constantly refer, were adopted without it being known how much their implementation would cost and who would finance them. Unfortunately, this uncertainty about the financing of the SDGs remains.

The recently published Report of the Secretary-General on Progress Towards Attaining the Sustainable Development Goals reminds us that it will take exceptional efforts and commitments to achieve a "rescue plan for people and planet" (United Nations, 2024). This is necessary at a time when many developing countries are facing disasters linked to climate change, the consequences of the COVID-19 pandemic and the war in Ukraine and the Middle East, rising foreign debt and inflation, among other challenges.

To achieve this, we need to increase funding for the SDGs, including for health, and reform the international financial architecture to make it resilient, equitable and accessible to all. The existing architecture, designed by the industrialized countries in the post-war period, has not lived up to the ambitions of the millennium development goals (MDGs). Its structural inequalities and inefficiencies hinder the achievement of international goals and have led to inadequate responses to the various crises (IISD, 2023).

2.10 Conclusions: Three Possible Scenarios for the Future of Global Health

2.10.1 Extension of the Current Status Quo

1. The proliferation of global health players, with a degree of juxtaposition and incoherence in their actions and, above all, the impossibility of effective and real coordination.
2. The conclusion of negotiations in the WHO on a pandemic treaty and the reform of the International Health Regulations (2005) without binding rules on substantive issues such as intellectual property and equity in access to products and technologies.

---

[5] The Third International Conference on Financing for Development, held in Addis Ababa, ended on 16 July 2015.

3. The idea that the WHO coordinates and governs the many players involved in global health.

Maintaining the status quo, i.e., responding or taking action (multilateral or national actors) as was done during the COVID-19 pandemic, would lead to another failure of global solidarity in the event of a new pandemic, to an apartheid in access to vaccines, diagnostics and treatments (as the WHO Director-General himself described it during COVID-19), and to the progressive erosion of multilateralism as a form of global health governance.

2.10.2   Global Health in the Hands of the Private Sector?

The scenario that favours the systematic entry of the private sector into health financing and management raises serious questions about how to guarantee equity and universal coverage in developing countries.

Whilst the private sector's involvement in managing climate change or in clean and more profitable technologies is obvious and can certainly be recognized, one might ask how the private sector can manage inequality in access to healthcare. For example, more environmentally friendly pharmaceutical technologies could be found, but if they are more expensive, they will only be accessible to a small number of people.

The growing involvement of the G7 in encouraging the private sector to play a greater role in the governance of global health is creating an imbalance and inequalities that are particularly problematic.

2.10.3   Regional Solutions

Given the interdependence of health technologies and pharmaceutical products, no country today is totally independent in the field of health, as demonstrated by the COVID-19 response.

Given the inability of the multilateral system to adopt global solutions, regional initiatives and solutions could provide a way out. These could include the regional manufacture of vaccines and medical supplies, the creation of regional medicines agencies with sanitary standards that promote regional health and production (the Latin American and Caribbean Medicines Agency—AMLAC-, proposed by certain Latin American countries, or the African Medicines Agency), as well as a regional approach to intellectual property standards, the use of the flexibilities in the TRIPS Agreement, cooperation and the strengthening of South–South cooperation.

This new regional dynamic could, at the same time, lead to a return to more equitable multilateral relations, in the interests and well-being of all.

References

Aldis, W. (2008). Health security as a public health concept: a critical analysis. *Health Policy and Planning, 23*(6), 369–375. https://doi.org/10.1093/heapol/czn030

Babacan, H. (2020). Public-private partnership for global health. In R. Haring et al. (Eds.), *Handbook of global health.*, ISBN: 978-3-030-05325-3. Springer 2021. https://citations.springernature.com. https://doi.org/10.1007/978-3-030-05325-3_117-1

Bass, E., & Russell, A. (2022a). Fix it or forget it. *Think Global Health.* 11 July 2022. https://www.thinkglobalhealth.org/article/fix-it-or-forget-it

Bass, E., & Russell, A. (2022b). Back from the Brink. *Think Global Health.* 6 October 2022.

BBC NEWS Afrique. (2023). Qu'est-ce que le groupe des BRICS et quels sont ses objectifs ? 21 August 2023 https://www.bbc.com/afrique/articles/clk1gy1dnn1o.

Bretton Woods Project. (2022). World Bank's commitment to private sector-led development casts doubt on effectiveness of new Pandemic Preparedness Fund, 21 July 2022. https://www.brettonwoodsproject.org/2022/07/world-banks-commitment-to-private-sector-led-development-casts-doubt-on-effectiveness-of-new-pandemic-preparedness-fund/.

BRICS Information Centre. (2011). BRICS health ministers' meeting: Beijing declaration. Beijing, China, 11 July 2011. http://www.brics.utoronto.ca/docs/110711-health.html.

BRICS Information Centre. (2012). Joint Communiqué of the BRICS member states on health, 22 May 2012. http://www.moh.gov.cn/publicfiles/business/htmlfiles/mohgjhzs/s3578/201205/54869.htm

Clark, H. (2023). Statement by Helen Clark former co-chair of the independent panel on pandemic preparedness and response opening segment of the UNGA high-level meeting on pandemic prevention, preparedness and response 20 September 2023, UNHQ, NY. https://www.helenclarknz.com/speeches-on-sustainable-development-gender-equality-and-climate-action/un-general-assembly-high-level-meeting-on-pandemic-prevention-preparedness-and-response.

Dentico, N. (2020). Ricchi e Buoni? le trame oscure del filantrocapitalismo, EMI 2020.

Drishti The Vision. (2019). Non-aligned movement (NAM), https://www.drishtiias.com/to-the-points/Paper2/non-aligned-movement-nam.

ECONOMIQUEMENT.FR. (2025). G7, G20, à quoi servent ces groupes des plus grandes puissances économiques ? https://www.economiquement.fr/dossier-56-g7-g20-groupes-grandes-puissances-economiques.html.

G7. (2022). Communiqué issued by the G7 health ministers on 20 May 2022, Berlin. https://www.g7germany.de/resource/blob/974430/2042058/5651daa321517b089cdccfaffd1e37a1/2022-05-20-g7-health-ministers-communique-data.pdf.

G7. (2023). Impact Investment Initiative for Global Health. https://www.mofa.go.jp/files/100507018.pdf.

Government of Spain. (2025). G20 El Grupo de los Veinte. https://www.tesoro.es/asuntos-internacionales/g20-el-grupo-de-los-veinte.

Harmer, A., et al. (2013). 'BRICS without straw'? A systematic literature review of newly emerging economies' influence in global health. *Global Health, 9,* 15. https://doi.org/10.1186/1744-8603-9-15

Heinrich-Böll-Stiftung. (2016). The G7 and G20 in the global governance landscape G20 fundamentals no. 2, October 2016. https://www.boell.de/sites/default/files/uploads/2016/11/fundamentals2_eng.pdf.

Hernández Zubizarreta, J. (2009). LAS EMPRESAS TRANSNACIONALES FRENTE A LOS DERECHOS HUMANOS: HISTORIA DE UNA ASIMETRIA NORMATIVA De la responsabilidad social corporativa a las redes contrahegemónicas transnacionales. ISBN: 978-84-89916-27-9.

IISD. (2023). Recommitting to finance the sustainable development goals, SDG knowledge hub. 28 June 2023. https://sdg.iisd.org/commentary/guest-articles/recommitting-to-finance-the-sustainable-development-goals/

Tagmatarchi Storeng, K., Puyvallée, A., & Stein, F. (2021). COVAX and the rise of the 'super public private partnership' for global health. *Global Public Health, 2021.* https://doi.org/10.108 0/17441692.2021.1987502

Kentikelenis, A. et al (2020). Softening the blow of the pandemic: will the International Monetary Fund and World Bank make things worse? *The Lancet,* Global Health, April 2020 https://www.thelancet.com/journals/langlo/article/PIIS2214-109X(20)30135-2/fulltext#%20.

Kickbusch. et al (2022). G7 measures to enhance global health equity and security, issue paper, 22 April 2022 . https://archive.think7.org/g7-measures-to-enhance-global-health-equity-and-security/.

Kolbert, E. (2018). Gospels of giving for the new gilded age: Are today's donor classes solving problems-or creating new ones?, The *New Yorker,* 20/8/2018 (bit.ly/20TFTYM).

Li, Y., Uribe, D., & Danish. (2023). *Reinvigorating the non-aligned movement for the post-COVID-19 Era,* Research Paper No. 179. Geneva: South Centre, 14 July 2023). https://www.southcentre.int/research-paper-179-14-july-2023/.

Liberation.fr. (2023). *Six nouveaux pays rejoignent les BRICS, le bloc des pays émergents* [archive], on *liberation.fr.*

Malpass, D. (2020). Remarks by David Malpass, President of the World Bank Group, at the G20 Finance Ministers' Conference Call on COVID-19. World Bank, 23 March 2020. https://www.worldbank.org/en/news/speech/2020/03/23/remarks-by-world-bank-group-president-david-malpass-on-g20-finance-ministers-conference-call-on-covid-19.

Marchal, B., Cavalli, A., & Kegels, G. (2009). Global health actors claim to support health system strengthening—is this reality or rhetoric? *PLoS Medicine, 6*(4), e1000059. https://doi.org/10.1371/journal.pmed.1000059

McBride, B., Hawkes, S., & Buse, K. (2019). Soft power and global health: The sustainable development goals (SDGs) era health agendas of the G7, G20 and BRICS. *BMC Public Health, 19,* 815. https://doi.org/10.1186/s12889-019-7114-5

McCoy, D. et al (2009). The Bill & Melinda Gates Foundation's grant-making programme for global health. https://doi.org/10.1016/S0140-6736(09)60571-7.

Moon, S., & Kickbusch, I. (2021). A pandemic treaty for a fragmented global polity, *Lancet* Public Health, June 2021. Available from HTTPS://WWW.SCIENCEDIRECT.COM/SCIENCE/ARTICLE/PII/S2468266721001031.

Permana, E. (2020). Países no alineados respaldan a la OMS y al multilateralismo, Agencia Anadolu, 05.05.2020 https://www.aa.com.tr/es/mundo/pa%C3%ADses-no-alineados-respaldan-a-la-oms-y-al-multilateralismo/1830284.

Prah Ruger, J. (2011). The changing role of the World Bank in Global Health. *American Journal of Public Health.* https://ajph.aphapublications.org. https://doi.org/10.2105/AJPH.2004.042002

Reich, R., Cordelli, C., & Bernholz, L. (2016). *Philanthropy in democratic societies: History, institutions, values.* The University of Chicago Press, University of Chicago.

Richter, J. (2004). *"Public-private partnerships and international health policy-making" how can public interests be safeguarded?* ISBN 951-724-464-9 Helsinki: Hakapaino Oy. https://um.fi/publications/-/asset_publisher/TVOLgBmLyZvu/content/elements-for-discussion-public-private-partnerships-and-international-health-policy-making.

Stuckler, D., Basu, S., & McKee, M. (2011). Global health philanthropy and institutional relationships: How should conflicts of interest be addressed? *PLoS Medicine, 8*(4), e1001020. https://doi.org/10.1371/journal.pmed.1001020

The Pandemic Fund. (2025). FAQ: Financial intermediary fund for pandemic prevention, preparedness and response. https://www.worldbank.org/en/topic/pandemics/brief/factsheet-financial-intermediary-fund-for-pandemic-prevention-preparedness-and-response.

Torchia, M., Calabrò, A., & Morner, M. (2015). Public-private partnerships in the health care sector: A systematic review of the literature. *Public Management Review, 17*(2), 236–261. https://www.tandfonline.com. https://doi.org/10.1080/14719037.2013.792380

TWN. (2015). The third financing for development conference in Addis Ababa: Failing to finance development? 2015. https://www.twn.my/title2/wto.info/2015/ti150717.htm

United Nations. (2015). Addis Ababa Action Agenda of the Third International Conference on Financing for Development, United Nations, New York, 2015. https://www.un.org/esa/ffd/publications/aaaa-outcome.html.

United Nations. (2023). Universal Health coverage: expanding our ambition for health and well-being in a post-COVID world. https://docs.un.org/en/A/RES/78/4

United Nations. (2024). Progress towards the sustainable development goals. Report of the Secretary-General.   https://unstats.un.org/sdgs/report/2024/The-Sustainable-Development-Goals-Report-2024.pdf.

United Nations News. (2021). COVID-19: New $50 billion initiative to end the pandemic and ensure global recovery, https://news.un.org/es/story/2021/06/1492752.

Velásquez G (2016). ¿ Qué remedios para la Organización Mundial de la Salud? una organización a la deriva, Le Monde Diplomatique, (Spanish edition), November 2016. https://mondiplo.com/que-remedios-para-la-organizacion-mundial-de-la.

Velásquez, G. (2023). *Where global health financing comes from and where it goes*, research paper no. 176. Geneva: South Centre, 29 March 2023). Available from https://www.southcentre.int/research-paper-176-29-march-2023/.

WEMOS, Eurodad. (2022). Collective civil society inputs in response to the World Bank Group's White Paper A Proposed Financial Intermediary Fund (FIF) for Pandemic Prevention, Preparedness and Response hosted by the World Bank. 17 May 2022. https://assets.nationbuilder.com/eurodad/pages/2957/attachments/original/1654272321/FIF_consultation_input_Wemos_and_Eurodad_including_endorsements.pdf?1654272321.

WHO. (2019). Thirteenth programme of work 2019–2023. https://iris.who.int/bitstream/handle/10665/324775/WHO-PRP-18.1eng.pdf?isAllowed=y&sequence=1.

WHO. (2021). G7 announces pledges of 870 million COVID-19 vaccine doses, of which at least half to be delivered by the end of 2021. Joint Press Release, Geneva, 13 June 2021. https://www.who.int/news/item/13-06-2021-g7-announces-pledges-of-870-million-covid-19-vaccine-doses-of-which-at-least-half-to-be-delivered-by-the-end-of-2021.

World Bank. (2022). New fund for pandemic prevention, preparedness and response formally established. Press Release, 9 September 2022. https://www.worldbank.org/en/news/press-release/2022/09/09/new-fund-for-pandemic-prevention-preparedness-and-response-formally-established.

World Bank. (2023). Brief July 20, 2023, FAQ: Pandemic Fund First Round of Funding Allocations https://www.worldbank.org/en/programs/financial-intermediary-fund-for-pandemic-prevention-preparedness-and-response-ppr-fif/brief/faq-pandemic-fund-first-round-of-funding-allocations?cq_ck=1689894483379.

Chapter 3
The Origins and Purpose of Global Health Financing

3.1 Introduction

Many of us believe, as Mariana Mazzucato mentioned in a book during the COVID-19 pandemic in 2020, that it was an opportunity to use the crisis "To understand how to do capitalism differently. This means rethinking the role of governments: instead of simply correcting market failures when they occur, they should be actively shaping and creating markets that generate sustainable and inclusive growth. They should also ensure that partnerships with publicly funded companies are driven by the public interest, not profit" (Mazzucato, 2022).

Mazzucato's optimism is tempered by her analysis that "the dominant role of business in public life has also led to a loss of confidence in what government alone can achieve. This has given rise to many problematic public-private partnerships, which prioritise the interests of business over those of the public. For example, it is well known that public-private partnerships in research and development often favour 'blockbusters' at the expense of drugs that are less commercially attractive but very important for public health, such as antibiotics and vaccines..." (Mazzucato, 2022).

Unfortunately, the management of COVID-19 in 2021 and 2022 confirmed that Mazzucato's concerns were well-founded, despite her warning: "Significant public funding of health innovation requires governments to be in the driving seat to ensure that prices are fair, patents are not abused, drug supply is guaranteed, and profits are reinvested in innovation rather than diverted to shareholders" (Mazzucato, 2022). Today, we know that prices were neither transparent nor fair, that the supply of vaccines was inequitable, and that the intellectual property exemption requested by

---

This chapter is largely taken from: Velásquez, G. (2023). Where does global health funding come from and where does it go?, Research Paper, No. 176, South Centre, Geneva. https://www.econstor.eu/handle/10419/278460.

© The Author(s), under exclusive license to Springer Nature Switzerland AG 2025
G. Velásquez, *Negotiating Global Health Policies*, SpringerBriefs in Public Health, https://doi.org/10.1007/978-3-031-99847-8_3

developing countries at the WTO came too late and was not equal to the problem. Nor do we know whether companies that have received large public subsidies (Mantilla & Barona, 2022) and made huge profits are reinvesting in innovation. According to second-quarter financial data recently released by the companies themselves, it is estimated that "Moderna has invoiced more than $6 billion in revenues to date, including $4.3 billion in net profits, representing a 69 percent margin on vaccine sales. Moderna expects to reach total vaccine sales of $20 billion by the end of 2021" (OXFAM, 2021a).

As long ago as 2020, some people were saying that "to be effective, the response to the current economic and health crisis must be guided by the values of international solidarity, multilateralism and equality" (Abbas, 2020). What we know today is that this has not been the case.

But the substantial public funding of vaccine producers is just one example of the "generosity" that certain governments can show at any given time. In this chapter, we want to go further and look at where the money that developed countries spend on global health comes from and where it goes.

We will see how, despite the fact that during major crises (HIV/AIDS, Ebola, COVID-19) the rhetoric of strengthening the WHO prevails, in practice the money goes to other institutions or new institutions or mechanisms are even created to manage the health crisis of the moment. We will also analyse what official development assistance (ODA) represents and how it is used in the health sector.

3.2   Context

In April 1945, at the Conference for the creation of the United Nations Organization (UNO) in San Francisco, representatives of Brazil and China proposed the creation of an international health organization and the convening of a conference to draft its constitution. A preparatory technical committee met in Paris from 18 March to 5 April 1946 and drafted proposals for a constitution in response to this initiative. The Conference on International Health, held in New York from 19 June to 22 July 1946, drafted and adopted the Constitution of the World Health Organization, which was signed on 22 July 1946 by representatives of 51 members of the United Nations and 10 other nations.

The Constitution came into force on 7 April 1948, when 26 of the 61 governments that had signed it ratified it (WHO, 2025a).

As Nirmalya Syam points out, the objectives of the WHO Constitution were very progressive and laid the foundations for addressing public health problems from a socio-economic and developmental perspective in order to strengthen health systems in countries that lacked them; it explicitly recognized the uneven development of public health. However, as Syam explains in his article, since the 1980s, this role of the WHO has been increasingly compromised by the emergence of new institutions and new funding mechanisms in the field of global health (Syam, 2023).

3.3 Original WHO Funding Model (1948–1998)

The original funding model of the WHO was based on contributions from member countries. These are assessed contributions and are "the dues countries pay in order to be a member of the Organization. The amount each Member State must pay is calculated relative to the country's wealth and population" (WHO, 2025b).

The scale of regular contributions that each of the 196 members and associate members must pay annually to the WHO is calculated by the United Nations,[1] mainly on the basis of the country's GDP and population. The World Health Assembly approves the budget every 2 years on the basis of the assessed contributions.

Regular assessed contributions are an essential source of funding for the organization, providing predictable funding, helping to minimize donor dependency and aligning resources with the programme budget.

Initially, since its creation in 1948, the WHO has relied on regular contributions from its Member States to finance its regular budget. A budget based mainly on regular contributions from the Member States made it possible, in principle, to set priorities independently and democratically, with the participation of the Member States.

However, regular contributions have fallen considerably as a percentage of the overall programme budget over the last 30 years, and now represent only 16 percent of the organization's funding (WHO, 2025c).

At the end of the 1980s (under the administration of H. Nakajima, from 1988 to 1998), the WHO World Health Assembly on the initiative of the United States and other industrialized countries agreed a policy of "zero real growth" in the recurrent budget (Krim, 1998; Merson & Inrig, 2018a). This policy remained in place for several decades, until the World Health Assembly in 2022. The WHO has therefore been forced to rely increasingly on raising additional voluntary contributions, known as "extra-budgetary funds" (EBFs). Between 1998 and 2003 (under the administration of Gro Harlem Brundtland), the real value of extra-budgetary funds exceeded the regular budget, something that had never happened before. All WHO programmes, with the exception of the Assembly and the Executive Board, received extra-budgetary funds (Vaughan JP et al., 1996).

Article 57 of the 1948 WHO Constitution states that "The Health Assembly, or the Board acting in its name and on its behalf, may accept and administer gifts and bequests made to the organization, provided that the conditions attached thereto are acceptable to the Health Assembly or the Board and consistent with the aims and policies of the organization".[2] This very general article does not specify the source of donations or limit their amount. This has allowed the organization to find itself today with the budget imbalance we have just mentioned (the organization's regular

---

[1] This is because the WHO is a specialized agency of the United Nations.
[2] Article 57 of the WHO Constitution.

assessed contributions represent only 16 percent of the total budget). Is it still possible to refer to it as a public international agency for global health management?

Given that Article 57 sets no limit on the amount that an individual donor may contribute, there is a risk that an entity, even a philanthropic one, could end up being the organization's main donor. This is the case of the Bill & Melinda Gates Foundation, which is currently the second largest contributor to the organization's budget.

3.4   Funding of WHO Regional Offices

The WHO has six regional offices located in Brazzaville, Cairo, Copenhagen, Manila, New Delhi and Washington, and they receive a share of the overall WHO budget each biennium, according to parameters that are regularly reviewed.

3.4.1   The Unique Case of the Americas Regional Office: Mixed Funding

The WHO Regional Office for the Americas, the Pan American Health Organization (PAHO) has a special, and in a sense, problematic status. This regional office was incorporated into PAHO, which was created in 1902 and already existed as a regional organization when the WHO was founded in 1948.

The budget of this regional office for the Americas comes from two sources: funds transferred from WHO headquarters in Geneva and contributions from each country in the region. The countries of the Americas must therefore pay a double contribution, one to the WHO in Geneva and the other directly to PAHO in Washington.

One might wonder why the countries of the Americas region pay a double financial contribution. We might also ask to what extent the weight of the American contribution to PAHO influences the implementation in the region of the recommendations and measures decided by all the member countries in Geneva.

3.5   Kofi Annan's Global Compact at the United Nations

In the United Nations system, public–private partnerships (PPPs) came into being at the end of the 1990s with the reform of the United Nations system launched by Secretary-General Kofi Annan. In response to resolution 55/215 "Towards global partnerships", the UN General Assembly asked the Secretary-General to "seek the views of all Member States on ways and means to enhance cooperation between the

United Nations and all relevant partners, in particular the private sector" (United Nations, 2001a). The introduction to the Secretary-General's report states that "over the past decade (...) the number of non-State actors interacting with the United Nations has increased (...), for example through consultations within governing bodies, procurement contracts and philanthropic fundraising activities" (United Nations (2001b). It also points out that "the number, diversity and influence of non-state actors have grown considerably over the past decade" and concludes that "special efforts are needed to ensure that cooperation with the business community and other non-state actors adequately reflects the composition of the organization and pays particular attention to the needs and priorities of developing countries" (Richter, 2004).

The purpose of the Global Compact is to encourage private sector companies to align their operations and strategies with universally accepted principles in the areas of human rights, labour, the environment and anti-corruption: "The Global Compact invites companies to embrace universal principles and to join with the United Nations. It has become an essential platform for the United Nations to engage effectively with the world's enlightened companies" (UN Global Compact, 2011). The Global Compact[3] invites companies to adopt, support and promulgate, within their sphere of influence, 10 principles in the areas of human rights, labour standards, the environment and anti-corruption (see Box 3.1).

Box 3.1 Principles of the United Nations Global Compact Initiative (UN Global Compact, 2025)
Human rights

- Principle 1: Businesses should support and respect the protection of internationally proclaimed human rights; and
- Principle 2: Ensure that they are not complicit in human rights abuses.

Work

- Principle 3: Businesses should respect freedom of association and effectively recognize the right to collective bargaining;
- Principle 4: The elimination of all forms of forced and compulsory labour;
- Principle 5: The effective abolition of child labour; and
- Principle 6: The elimination of discrimination in respect of employment and occupation.

---

[3] The UN Global Compact involves the following key UN agencies:
Office of the United Nations High Commissioner for Human Rights (OHCHR)
United Nations Environment Programme
International Labour Organisation
United Nations Development Programme
United Nations Industrial Development Organization
United Nations Office on Drugs and Crime
UN-Women: United Nations Entity for Gender Equality and the Empowerment of Women
See: http://www.unglobalcompact.org/AboutTheGC/.

Environment

– Principle 7: Companies are encouraged to adopt a precautionary approach to environmental challenges;
– Principle 8: Take initiatives to promote greater environmental responsibility; and
– Principle 9: Encourage the development and dissemination of environmentally friendly technologies.

Fighting corruption

– Principle 10: Businesses are encouraged to combat corruption in all its forms, including extortion and bribery.

During the tenure of Margaret Chan as Director-General of the World Health Organization (2007–2017), extensive deliberations took place concerning the role of non-State actors in global health governance. Although certain aspects of the proposed reform were implemented, the specific role of private sector entities remained insufficiently defined.

It is noteworthy that the WHO does not participate in the United Nations Global Compact, despite being one of the UN agencies most extensively engaged in public–private partnerships. This omission appears paradoxical, particularly given that none of the initiative's 10 core principles explicitly address public health or the fundamental right to healthcare access.

3.6 Progressive Privatization of the WHO: Increasing Reliance on Private, Philanthropic and Voluntary Public Contributions Beyond the Core Budget

The World Health Organization wasn't greatly influenced by the commercial sector until 1998. The Member States demanded that all normative programmes be fully funded by the regular budget from Member State payments, and that the normal public budget should make up at least half of the organization's budget (Velásquez, 2014).

PDPs can be considered to be the precursors of the WHO Special Programme for Research and Training in Tropical Diseases (TDR). With assistance from the World Bank, the United Nations Development Programme (UNDP), and the United Nations Children's Fund (UNICEF), the WHO established the TDR in 1975. Its goals were to: establish research priorities; foster collaboration with national institutions and other governmental and non-governmental organizations to coordinate research in this area; promote and intensify research on tropical diseases, keeping in mind that these activities should primarily be conducted in endemic countries; and mobilize extra-budgetary resources to further these goals.[4] The TDR was established primarily as a collaborative initiative involving public donors, co-sponsoring organizations and the governments of disease-endemic countries, all represented within an independent, council-like governance structure. The programme's research priorities were determined by a scientific committee of experts, which was responsible for selecting research projects for funding and for evaluating the progress of scientific working groups and technical personnel, with participation from representatives of endemic countries (UNICEF/UNDP/World Bank/WHO Special Programme for Research and Training in Tropical Diseases & World Health Organization, 2007).

Several practices introduced by TDR during the 1970s and 1980s laid the groundwork for models later adopted by Product Development Partnerships (PDPs). Notably, TDR established a global network of academic institutions to evaluate the efficacy of pharmaceutical products in treating tropical diseases. In this regard, TDR can be considered a forerunner of PDPs—and arguably, a contributing factor to some of the contemporary challenges in global health governance.

Director-General Brundtland said in her first address to the WHA that in order to fulfil the mandate assigned to her. "We must reach out to the private sector (…) The private sector has an important role to play both in technology development and the provision of services. We must have honest and positive relationships with business and the private sector, understanding the areas in which our tasks may complement one another and where they diverge. I encourage industry to participate in a discussion about the main concerns we face" (WHO, 1998).

Due to the financial difficulties of WHO brought on by the developed countries' refusal to increase its regular budget and its lack of credibility in the last years of Director-General Nakajima's administration, the Brundtland administration turned to the private sector for assistance in resolving these issues. Specifically, it introduced high-level personnel from multinational pharmaceutical companies into the WHO.[5]

What Buse and Walt refer to as "growing disillusionment with the UN and its agencies" had a significant impact on Brundtland's invitation to the private sector. Partnerships were formed to address specific and limited challenges as a direct result of concerns about the UN's efficacy, including mounting evidence of overlapping mandates and agency competition (Buse & Walt, 2000).

During the 5-year tenure of the Brundtland administration at the World Health Organization, there was a significant increase in the number of public–private partnerships (PPPs) and product development partnerships (PDPs) across various areas of WHO's work, as well as within broader international public health efforts. Many of these partnerships, particularly those focused on innovation and access to medicines, established their own advisory structures. In certain instances, these bodies

---

[4] In May 1974, the Twenty-Seventh World health Assembly adopted resolution WHA 27.52, calling for increased research on tropical parasitic diseases.

[5] This is the case of Michael Scholtz, former marketing director of SmithKline Beecham Biologicals, appointed by Brundtland as Assistant Director-General (ADG) for drugs.

may operate independently of—or even in divergence from—the WHO's formal governing entities, namely the Executive Board and the World Health Assembly.

Brundtland's engagement with the private sector proved to be highly effective. When she assumed the role of Director-General, the WHO programme budget for the 1998–1999 biennium stood at $1.8 billion. By the end of her tenure in 2003, this figure had risen to $2.8 billion, largely due to an increase in voluntary contributions from both public and private sector sources. This pattern of reliance on voluntary funding has not only continued under subsequent WHO leadership but has also intensified over time (Buse & Walt, 2000).

The WHO has a number of PPPs, particularly, but not exclusively, in the field of medicines for diseases such as trachoma (Pfizer), lymphatic filariasis (SmithKline Beecham), sleeping sickness (Hoechst Hoest) and onchocerciasis (Merck), to name but a few (Reich, 2002).

3.7   Official Development Assistance for Health

In the last year for which data was available (2018), health financing in countries that benefited from official development assistance (ODA) accounted for only 1.5 percent of total health financing available in developing countries. In other words, 98.5 percent of this expenditure is financed by national resources in these countries. (OECD, 2020).

Health aid to developing countries reported by the Organization for Economic Co-operation and Development (OECD) includes, in addition to the traditional bilateral cooperation agencies, the United States Agency for International Development (USAID), the British agency (DFID), the Swedish agency (SIDA), the German agency (GIZ), the funds intended for the Global Fund, the Global Alliance for Vaccines (GAVI) and the International Development Association (IDA).

According to OECD data:

1. International aid accounts for just 1.5 percent of total healthcare expenditure in developing countries.
2. Half of international health aid is spent on purchasing medicines from industries located mainly in donor countries (OECD, 2020).

Official development assistance to the health sector peaked in 2017 at US$24.4 billion, but fell by to US$22.2 billion in 2018.

The top three donors, the United States, the Global Fund and the United Kingdom, accounted for 60 percent of health aid in 2018, while the top 15 donors accounted for 90 percent of the total aid.

More than half of the aid from developed countries goes to HIV/AIDS, malaria and tuberculosis, and more than half of aid to health went to sub-Saharan Africa in 2018. Aid to health declined for several of the largest donors between 2017 and 2018.

A report published by the World Bank and the WHO before the COVID-19 pandemic already highlighted the fact that half the world has no access to essential health services, that 100 million people are driven into extreme poverty by health-care costs, and that a large number of households fall into poverty because they have to pay for healthcare out of their own pockets (World Bank & WHO, 2017).

The report makes it clear that health funding efforts must be stepped up urgently, while noting that several major health donors, including The Global Fund, the U.S. President's Emergency Plan for AIDS Relief (PEPFAR) and GAVI Alliance, are transferring responsibility for funding and implementing programmes to national governments in developing countries (McDonough & Rodriguez, 2020).

To ensure the effectiveness of the limited development aid allocated to low- and middle-income countries, it is essential that the pricing of essential medicines reflects a reasonable correlation with their actual development and production costs. The global response to the COVID-19 pandemic—particularly the widespread vaccination efforts and the shortcomings of the COVAX initiative—highlights critical issues in this regard. Due to the inadequacies of COVAX, many developing countries were compelled to purchase vaccines directly from pharmaceutical companies at significant financial cost.[6]

Analyses indicate that the leading mRNA vaccines, developed by Pfizer/BioNTech and Moderna with approximately $8.3 billion in public investment, could be produced for as little as $1.20 per dose. In contrast, the average cost of vaccines supplied through COVAX was nearly five times higher. Furthermore, COVAX failed to deliver sufficient quantities of vaccines within the necessary time frame, primarily because wealthier nations secured the majority of available doses by paying inflated prices (Oxfam, 2021b). This raises a critical question: is it justifiable to allocate development aid towards purchasing health technologies at prices significantly exceeding their production costs?

3.8   The Establishment of Parallel Organizations in the Health Sector

Independent health bodies operating outside the WHO framework have been established as a result of discussions and actions undertaken by WHO Member States since 1996. The reputation of the WHO as a global health organization has suffered as a result of this strategy (Velásquez, 2022).

---

[6] According to OXFAM, Moderna and Pfizer/BioNTech overcharged governments to the tune of 41 billion dollars.

3.8.1   UNAIDS 1996

Jonathan Mann, the director of the Global Programme on AIDS (GPA), promoted a broad strategy that took into account social, economic and human rights factors in order to manage the AIDS pandemic. Hiroshi Nakajima, the director-general of the WHO, promoted a biomedical strategy. Mann decided to step down in 1994 as a result of this (Merson & Inrig, 2018b). In 1996, the donors withdrew from the WHO programme, which at the time had the largest financial resources and was addressing the largest health issue facing the world, after the quick appointment of American Michael Merson to replace Jonathan Mann failed to allay their mistrust of the WHO's financial management.

After 2 years of discussion and debate, UNAIDS was founded in 1994–1995 under the leadership of Peter Piot (Velásquez, 2020).

This precedent could be used to support the current argument that an independent body from the WHO is required to prevent and prepare for pandemics in the future. Indeed, in certain discussions surrounding the proposed pandemic treaty, there have been suggestions that negotiations should take place outside the framework of the WHO (Moon & Kickbusch, 2021). However, such an approach would be misguided. Rather than creating parallel structures, efforts should focus on reinforcing the WHO's role and capacity as the leading global public health authority (Velásquez, 2020).

3.8.2   From the Expanded Programme on Immunization to the GAVI Partnership

The Expanded Programme on Immunization (EPI) was created by the WHO in 1974 to develop and extend immunization programmes worldwide (Keja et al., 1988).

A decade after the launch of the Expanded Programme on Immunization (EPI), the World Health Organization (WHO) established a standardized immunization schedule in 1984 for the initial set of EPI vaccines: oral polio vaccine, measles, diphtheria-tetanus-pertussis (DTP), and Bacillus Calmette-Guerin(BCG). Over time, this schedule was expanded to include additional vaccines such as hepatitis B (Hep B), yellow fever in endemic regions, and the conjugate vaccine against *Haemophilus influenzae* type b (Hib) in countries with a high disease burden (Jamison et al., 2006).

Every WHO Member State had a national immunization programme by the end of the 1990s, complete with a list of required immunizations based on WHO guidelines. With UNICEF's active guidance, developing country governments achieved notable advancements: "By 1990, 108 countries (43 percent of all children) had DTP3 coverage levels greater than 80 percent, and fewer than 10 percent of children lived in countries with under 50 percent coverage" (Burton et al., 2009). The EPI is without doubt one of the most effective initiatives of WHO in collaboration with UNICEF.

Tore Godal,[7] the TDR Director, withdrew the immunization programme from WHO and was named director of a new alliance known as "GAVI" at the beginning of the Brundtland administration, which was known to advocate for the private sector's participation in health initiatives. What led to the removal from the WHO of a successful programme that was overseen by WHO personnel and supported by another UN agency?

Several nations, UNICEF, WHO, the World Bank, the Bill & Melinda Gates Foundation, the vaccine industry, public health organizations, and non-governmental organizations joined together to form GAVI as a public–private partnership. GAVI was established with a grant from the Bill & Melinda Gates Foundation and has since received funding from nine nations as well as various private donors. According to ReliefWeb (2003), its total commitments in 2003 were US$1 billion, which was more than the WHO's whole regular budget at the time.[8] GAVI's budget for 2021–2025 is estimated at $21.4 billion (GAVI, 2025).

3.8.3   The Global Fund to Fight AIDS, Tuberculosis and Malaria

As a public–private partnership, the Global Fund seeks to raise money and mobilize support for the three diseases included in its name. The Global Fund was established in 2002 and is a member of the "new generation" of global health actors, fusing the knowledge of private industry and civil society with that of bilateral and multilateral organizations (Hanefeld, 2014).

Mrs. Brundtland attempted to persuade the developed nations to approve an increase in the regular budget, which had been governed by the zero-growth rule since the late 1980s, during the first 2 years of her term. The Brundtland administration looked at ways to raise more money for the organization after failing to get an increase in the regular budget. This gave rise to the notion of establishing a sizable worldwide fund that would be funded by the voluntarily donated funds of many developed nations. At first, this was an internal mechanism intended to support the WHO budget rather than a distinct fund for the organization.

The establishment of a global fund was suggested by Kofi Annan and Brundtland during the G8 meetings in Okinawa, Japan, in 2000, and Genoa, Italy, in July 2001. The establishment of the Global Fund as a separate entity from the WHO was announced in January 2002. Based on data supplied by the Global Fund itself:

---

[7] Tore Godal, a Norwegian, was one of the protagonists who convinced former Norwegian Prime Minister Brundtland to run for the WHO. After the election, Tore Godal imposed his Australian wife, Anne Kern, as assistant to the director-general and succeeded in pushing through the EPI to create the public–private partnership that came to be known as the GAVI Alliance.

[8] The WHO regular budget for 2002–2003 was $846.6 million.

As a partnership of governments, civil society, technical agencies, the private sector and people affected by the diseases, the Global Fund pools the world's resources to invest strategically in programmes to end AIDS, TB and malaria as public health threats. Since our creation, more than US$65 billion has been disbursed in the fight against HIV, TB and malaria and for programmes to strengthen systems for health across more than 155 countries, including regional grants, making us one of the largest funders of global health (The Global Fund, 2025).

3.8.4 Unitaid

Following an initiative proposed by Presidents Jacques Chirac and Luiz Ignacio Lula da Silva, Unitaid was created in September 2006 in the margins of the United Nations General Assembly under the patronage of UN Secretary-General Kofi Annan, with representatives from the five founding countries (France, Brazil, Norway, Chile and the United Kingdom) (Simon & De Lemos, 2006).

In February 2006, at the "Paris Conference" organized by France and Brazil, a number of nations agreed to levy a fee on airplane tickets as a form of solidarity. The funds would be utilized to buy medications to treat tuberculosis, HIV/AIDS and malaria. Unitaid would also be a tool for reducing costs and accelerating access to medications in underdeveloped nations by mobilizing steady and predictable funding resources. The WHO would host Unitaid, an independent organization that would support current organizations battling these three key diseases.

In France, the tax on airline tickets was adopted by the law of 22 December 2005 and came into force on 1 July 2006. When Unitaid was set up, it was estimated that France alone could contribute $220 million a year to the purchase of medicines by supporting the national pharmaceutical policies of beneficiary countries (Simon & De Lemos, 2006).

Fifteen years after its creation, Unitaid is today, as stated on its website: "a global health agency dedicated to finding innovative solutions to prevent, diagnose and treat diseases faster, cheaper and more effectively in low- and middle-income countries. Our work includes funding initiatives to tackle major diseases such as HIV/AIDS, malaria and tuberculosis, as well as HIV-related co-infections and co-morbidities such as cervical cancer and hepatitis C, and cross-cutting areas such as fever management" (Unitaid, 2025).

Although it is independent and has its own management bodies, this creative and vibrant agency is nonetheless housed by the WHO. Donors have contributed over $3 billion to Unitaid since its founding in 2006. France, the United Kingdom, Norway, the Bill & Melinda Gates Foundation, Brazil, Spain, the Republic of Korea and Chile are the primary donors of Unitaid.

Innovative financing has been an important source of revenue, in particular the solidarity tax on airline tickets introduced by France, which was subsequently adopted by other countries (Cameroon, Chile, Congo, Guinea, Madagascar, Mali,

Mauritius, Niger and the Republic of Korea). However, air ticket taxes have not been adopted by the countries with the most air traffic, as the founders of Unitaid had expected.

3.8.5   The Medicines Patent Pool

The World Trade Organization (WTO), the World Intellectual Property Organization (WIPO), the WHO,[9] a representative of the UK aid agency (DFID), a representative of Médecins Sans Frontières' (MSF) Access to Medicines Campaign, and a representative of Knowledge Ecology International (KEI) participated in a series of meetings organized in 2008 and 2009 at Unitaid's initiative with the goal of establishing a patent community to expedite access to medications in developing countries.

The WHO and the Unitaid Secretariat, which championed the proposal, were clear from the start that the patent pool would promote both mandatory and voluntary licensing. In 2008, the WHO was explicitly tasked with promoting the "full" use of the flexibilities of the WTO TRIPS Agreement, particularly compulsory licensing, as outlined in World Health Assembly Resolution 61.21 ("Global Strategy and Plan of Action on Public Health, Innovation and Intellectual Property") and subsequent ones. WTO and WIPO representatives opted to stop attending Unitaid-organized meetings, claiming that it was outside their organizations' purview to advocate for or suggest the issuance of compulsory licences. MSF and KEI delegates agreed with Unitaid and WHO's stance. The UK Government envoy stated that his government had rejected the establishment of a body to support compulsory licensing after over 2 years of discussions.[10]

In order to increase access to reasonably priced therapies in low- and middle-income countries through voluntary licensing, Unitaid finally established the Medicines Patent Pool (MPP) in 2010. As long as the WHO's support of the use of compulsory licensing, as required by numerous resolutions, remained consistent and transparent, this institution may prove beneficial. Unfortunately, due to the WHO's so-called "tripartite" collaboration (WHO, WTO and WIPO), this has not been the case in recent years.

According to a Unitaid financial report, Unitaid has invested approximately US$60 million in the MPP since its creation (Unitaid, 2017).

---

[9] The author served as the WHO representative for the effort to establish a pharmaceutical patent pool at all of the 2008 and 2009 sessions.

[10] As the Director of the WHO Medicines Programme, the author participated in these negotiations.

3.8.6   Coalition for Epidemic Preparedness Innovations (CEPI)

According to information provided by CEPI, "... is an innovative partnership between public, private, philanthropic and civil organisations. Its mission is to accelerate the development of vaccines and other biologic countermeasures against epidemic and pandemic threats so they can be accessible to all people in need" (CEPI, 2017).

CEPI adopted a $3.5 billion plan over the period 2021–2022 to put an end to the COVID-19 pandemic. "Compared with the trillions lost to COVID-19, at $3.5 billion this plan is not only value for money, it's exactly what the world needs to ensure our children never again face the hardship and loss we've had to endure from COVID-19", said CEPI Director Richard Hatchett (CEPI, 2025).

Within a few months, this public–private collaboration outside of the primary international health body—the WHO—was granted access to these funds, which amounted to nearly the WHO budget for 2 years.

3.8.7   COVAX: 2021

A global partnership known as ACT Accelerator created a funding mechanism for COVID-19 vaccinations (also known as COVAX) in June 2020. The GAVI Alliance, WHO, and the Coalition for Epidemic Preparedness Innovation (CEPI), which was established in Davos in 2017, are co-leaders of this mechanism (GAVI, 2020).

Globally, the introduction of COVAX elicited overwhelmingly supportive responses, especially from Southern nations worried about fair access to upcoming vaccinations. No one was able to stop the industrialized nations and big pharmaceutical companies from ignoring the promises made, which led to the COVAX mechanism being questioned a year after it was established (Velásquez, 2021).

COVAX set out to provide vaccines to every nation on an equal basis at the onset of the epidemic. Regretfully, it fell short of half of its 2021 goal of delivering 2 billion doses (Taylor, 2021). In October 2021, an open letter to G20 leaders reported that low- and middle-income countries had administered four doses per 100 people, while high- and low-income countries had administered 133 doses per 100 people. Using the term "unequal access to vaccines" to highlight the scope of this ethical failing, the WHO Director-General referred to this failure as "vaccine apartheid" and made a clear analogy to South Africa's system of institutionalized racial segregation (WHO, 2021).

3.8.8   The "WHO Foundation"

"I am pleased to announce that this year will see the creation of the WHO Foundation, which will enable us to generate funding from hitherto untapped sources",[11] the Director-General remarked at the conclusion of a lengthy speech to the 72nd World Health Assembly in May 2019. The majority of participants were unaware of this revelation. The organization's governing bodies have never debated the establishment of a WHO Foundation, and neither the Executive Board nor the General Assembly has had a chance to vote on the matter.

However, in May 2020, the WHO welcomed the creation of the new foundation: "The World Health Organization (WHO) welcomes the creation of the WHO Foundation, an independent grant-making entity, that will support the Organization's efforts to address the most pressing global health challenges" (WHO, 2020).

Member countries were not consulted, nor give their approval for this significant and unprecedented adjustment in the organization's funding. "New forms of financing are being defined that may alter governance in a way that is directly contrary to the very objectives of public health", the Geneva Health Files state. Despite the concerns expressed by civil society actors, they were adopted and standardized without sufficient consultation with WHO Member States (Patnaik, 2021).

The WHO Director thanked Thomas Zeltner, who was then the Chairman of the WHO Executive Board and is currently the founder and Chairman of the Foundation's Board, for taking the initiative to create the WHO Foundation: "Today's announcement is the culmination of more than two years of preparation and hard work by countless individuals and partner organizations. I would like to thank Professor Thomas Zeltner for spearheading this incredible adventure and founding the organization" (WHO, 2020).

According to Mr Zeltner, "We have to create a healthier, more equitable future for everyone. By investing in 8 billion lives and by using a flexible, innovative, partnership-driven approach, our goal is to overcome the health challenges of today and ensure healthy lives tomorrow" (WHO Foundation, 2020). It would be important to know what the "flexible approach" to which Thomas Zeltner refers consists of.

The WHO Foundation states on its website that: "The World Health Organization (WHO) plays a unique role in leading the global health ecosystem, developing guidelines and technical tools to prevent and treat disease, and acting as a convener at the country level with an unparalleled level of trust. The crises of the 21st century, in particular the COVID-19 crisis, have highlighted the inequality of access to effective and affordable healthcare, and the indispensable role of the WHO. However, the WHO does not have sufficient resources to fulfil its mandate. And, beyond funding, its vision cannot be achieved by the public sector alone. *The WHO Foundation was established as an independent Swiss foundation, affiliated to but independent of WHO*, to raise new resources from philanthropists, foundations, corporations and

---

[11] Opening speech by the Director-General at the World Health Assembly, May 2019.

individuals to support its mission: to promote global health, ensure global security and serve the vulnerable".[12] (emphasis added).

In order to raise money for the WHO, the new WHO Foundation was established. Otherwise, there could have been conflicts of interest, as demonstrated by Nestlé's recent $2 million donation.

But it is not surprising that these donations have been made. Anil Soni clearly stated why the organization was established when he was named head of the Foundation. "We will have a new set of operational conditions that are more flexible in terms of company engagement, which is part of our raison d'être. Although there are typically exceptions, some industries will be off-limits since it's crucial for the WHO to be clear that it's not working with the tobacco and armaments industries".

For other industries and companies, we will actively seek to collaborate, and we will do so by following ethical guidelines that we will make public... (Patnaik, 2021) (paraphrased).

WHO Foundation is an independent grant-making foundation that is unique in the area of world health. WHO Foundation's role is to support the World Health Organization's (WHO's) mission both directly and by supporting WHO's network of partners on the ground. WHO Foundation is a force for new and better collective solutions. It brings together donors, world health professionals and the WHO network, to create partnerships that drive innovative actions to address the most pressing health challenges of today and tomorrow (Office of International Geneva, 2025).

The primary concern with this foundation is the extent of change in the way public international organizations are financed. However, one may also wonder how the funding will come from public or private donations to the WHO. To what extent does the allocation of funds for WHO activities depend on an "independent foundation" that receives a portion of the public agency's funding?

3.8.9   The WHO Working Group on Sustainable Financing

A working group on sustainable funding for the WHO was established as a result of the organization's insufficient budget issues. The WHA organized this group, which convened seven times between April 2021 and April 2022. They decided at their most recent meeting to deliver a draft conclusion and recommendations to the 75th WHA in May 2022. By going back to a regular public budget that was funded by member nations, the goal was to set the groundwork for funding that was democratic and sustainable and in accordance with the original WHO standards.

The 75th World Health Assembly adopted the following decision on financing:

The Seventy-fifth World Health Assembly, having considered the report of the Working Group on Sustainable Financing, including its associated recommendations,

---

[12] WHO Foundation https://who.foundation/.

Decided:

(1) to adopt the recommendations of the Working Group on Sustainable Financing, contained

in Annex 4; and

(2) to request the Director-General to put in place measures to ensure the implementation of

those recommendations.

With regard to the increase in the regular budget, Annex (e) of the Recommendations states: "that the Seventy-fifth World Health Assembly, recognizing the important role of assessed contributions in sustainably financing the Organization, requests the Secretariat to develop budget proposals, through the regular budget cycle, for an increase of assessed contributions to contribute to financial sustainability of WHO and with its aspiration to reach a level of 50 percent of the 2022–2023 base budget by the biennium 2030–2031, while aiming to achieve this by the biennium 2028–2029" (WHO, 2022).

The WHO's working group on sustainable financing, headed by German delegate Bjorn Kummel, made recommendations that were adopted at the WHA as a result of the COVID-19 debate. One of these recommendations was to create budget proposals as part of the regular budget cycle that would gradually increase contributions from the organization's regular budget until they represented the organization's budget during the 2028–2029 biennium. As previously stated, only 16 percent of the organization's budget is now allocated to the WHO's regular, or public, budget (WHO, 2022).

In January 2022, in a book published by Springer and widely distributed, the South Centre stated that: "In order to progressively restore the public character of the organization, mechanisms should be defined and put in place to control at least 51 percent of the budget, over a period of, say, 7 years. This means that regular compulsory contributions from Member States should represent at least 51 percent of the agency's total budget" (Velásquez, 2022).

This decision by the WHA to increase the organization's regular budget, which had been frozen and constrained to zero growth since the early 1980s[13] (Reddy et al., 2018), described as "historic" by several observers, contrasts with the recent announcement of the creation of a multi-billion dollar fund at the World Bank for the prevention of pandemics (World Bank, 2022).

---

[13] Reddy, S, Mazhar S., Lencucha R state that "In the early 1980s, the WHA introduced a 'zero-real growth policy' for the regular budget. This policy froze membership dues (i.e. assessed contributions) in real dollar terms so that only inflation and exchange rates would influence membership assessment adjustments. In 1993, the WHA voted for a more stringent budgetary policy, moving the organisation from 'zero real growth' to 'zero nominal growth for assessed contributions'".

3.9   Conclusions

Only a small portion of the money that developing nations invest in bolstering their healthcare systems comes from development aid. But not all of this money ends up in developing nations directly; instead, it is distributed through public–private partnerships and other organizations like the World Bank FIF, CEPI, COVAX, the WHO Foundation, and The Global Fund. Roughly half of the funding is designated for the acquisition of medications and vaccines made in a select few of the 15 donor nations.

The industrialized nations favour and are attempting to impose global health management administered by public–private consortiums created by these nations, as evidenced by the way COVID-19 was managed by CEPI, COVAX, the WHO Foundation and the World Bank's FIF. The WHO will serve as a non-voting observer and offer technical support to the public–private consortia that will make the choices, since it has been authorized to symbolically boost its public budget.

Although the WHO is described in the text as coordinating and governing, in reality, its role is limited to providing technical advice and monitoring decision-making.

Since the "WHO Foundation" has never received approval from the WHO regulatory bodies, its mission is unclear, and the procedures for avoiding conflicts of interest are not well defined.

Will the G7 and G20 take advantage of their power and impose to other countries their vision of managing global health?

In conclusion, the following issue may be raised: how can the preservation of human rights, the defence of shared public goods, and the public interest be preserved in the planning, prevention and reaction to present and future pandemics?

The role of the WHO should be strengthened as a result of the COVID-19 pandemic, according to recent international discussions, the World Health Assembly in 2022, and the G7 and G20 reports. In this regard, the World Health Assembly's decision to progressively raise the assessed contributions to 50% of the public contributions by 2028–2029 makes sense. The organization's regular public budget would only see a 1.2 billion dollar increase in total donations, which is somewhat confusing when contrasted to the several billions that the methods and entities discussed in this chapter will or hope to manage.

We have witnessed how access to vaccines, diagnostics and treatments were not guaranteed by international solidarity. The necessity for a legally enforceable international treaty on pandemics was brought to the attention of the world community by the COVID-19 issue. Amid all of this chaos, Russia began an irrational and expensive war against Ukraine, and the Atlantic Alliance has entered an arms race that might potentially redirect funds for much needed medical treatment to the acquisition of weapons. Strengthening the public health sector, including the WHO, and the resources that are now distributed across numerous organizations and processes that fracture rather than improve the coherence of the global health system is obviously necessary for effective preparation for future pandemics.

References

Abbas, M. Z. (2020). *Practical implications of vaccine nationalism: A short-sighted and risky approach in response to COVID-19*, Research Paper No. 124. Geneva: South Centre, November 2020. https://www.southcentre.int/research-paper-124-november-2020/.

Burton, A., et al. (2009). WHO and UNICEF estimates of national infant immunization coverage: methods and processes. *Bull World Health Organ, 87*(7), 535–541. https://doi.org/10.2471/blt.08.053819

Buse, K., & Walt, G. (2000). Global public-private partnerships: Part I—a new development in health? *Bulletin of the World Health Organization, 78*(4), 549–561.

CEPI. (2017). CEPI officially launched, 18th January 2017. https://cepi.net/cepi-officially-launched.

CEPI. (2025). Developing pandemic-busting vaccines in 100 days by Dr Richard Hatchett. https://cepi.net/100-days.

GAVI. (2020). The Bill & Melinda Gates Foundation. https://www.gavi.org/operating-model/gavis-partnership-model/gates-foundation.

GAVI. (2025). Donor contributions: 2021–2025. https://www.gavi.org/investing-gavi/funding/current-period-2021-2025.

Hanefeld, J. (2014). The global fund to fight AIDS, Tuberculosis and Malaria: 10 years on NIH. *Clinical Medicine, 14*(1), 54–57. https://doi.org/10.7861/clinmedicine.14-1-54

Jamison, D. T., et al. (2006). *Disease control priorities in developing countries* (2nd ed.). World Bank and Oxford University Press. http://hdl.handle.net/10986/7242.

Keja, K., et al. (1988). Expanded programme on immunization. *World Health Stat Q, 41*(2), 59–63. https://pubmed.ncbi.nlm.nih.gov/3176515/

Krim, M. (1998). Jonathan Mann 1947–1998. *Nature Medicine, 4*, 1101. https://doi.org/10.1038/2592

Mantilla, K. K., & Barona, C. C. (2022). *COVID-19 vaccines as global public goods: Between life and profit*, Research Paper No. 154. Geneva: South Centre, 9 May 2022). https://www.south-centre.int/research-paper-154-9-may-2022/.

Mazzucato, M. (2022). *No desaprovechemos esta crisis. Lecciones de la COVID-19*. ED. Galaxia Gutemberg: Barcelona, 2022.

McDonough, A., & Rodriguez, D. C. (2020). How donors support civil society as government accountability advocates: A review of strategies and implications for transition of donor funding in global health. *Globalization and Health, 16*, 110. https://doi.org/10.1186/s12992-020-00628-6

Merson, M., & Inrig, S. (2018a). End of the global programme on AIDS and the launch of UNAIDS. In: *The AIDS pandemic: Searching for a global response* (Springer, 2018). https://doi.org/10.1007/978-3-319-47133-4_16

Merson M and Inrig S (2018b). The Resignation of Jonathan Mann. In: *The AIDS pandemic: Searching for a global response*. Springer, . https://doi.org/10.1007/978-3-319-47133-4_7

Moon, S., & Kickbusch, I. (2021). A pandemic treaty for a fragmented global polity. *Lancet* Public Health, June 2021. https://www.sciencedirect.com/science/article/pii/s2468266721001031.

OECD. (2020). Aid spent on health: ODA data on donors, sectors, recipients. Factsheet, 24 July 2020. https://devinit.org/resources/aid-spent-health-oda-data-donors-sectors-recipients/.

Office of International Geneva. (2025). Who's who? WHO Foundation. https://www.geneve-int.ch/whoswho/who-foundation.

OXFAM. (2021a). Despite Big Pharma's profits from COVID-19 vaccines, the taxes they pay are low. OXFAM Intermon, 15 September 2021. https://www.oxfamintermon.org/es/nota-de-prensa/beneficios-grandes-farmac%C3%A9uticas-vacuna-covid19-pagan-bajos-impuestos.

OXFAM. (2021b). Vaccine monopolies make cost of vaccinating the world against COVID at least 5 times more expensive than it could be. 29 July 2021. https://www.oxfam.org/en/press-releases/vaccine-monopolies-make-cost-vaccinating-world-against-covid-least-5-times-more.

Patnaik, P. (2021). A hole in the firewall: The WHO Foundation & WHO; Green shoots for TRIPS Waiver Talks? Geneva Health Files, Newsletter No. 50, April 2021. https://genevahealthfiles. substack.com/p/a-hole-in-the-firewall-the-who-foundation.

Reddy, S., Mazhar, S., & Lencucha, R. (2018). The financial sustainability of the World Health Organization and the political economy of global health governance: a review of funding proposals. Global Health, 14, 119. (2018). https://doi.org/10.1186/s12992-018-0436-8

Reich, M. R. (Ed.). (2002). Public-private partnerships for public health (Harvard series on population and international health). Harvard Center for Population and Development Studies, Distributed by Harvard University Press.

ReliefWeb. (2003). Press release: Over 1 billion committed to immunize world's poorest children. 15 July 2003. https://reliefweb.int/report/angola/over-1-billion-committed-immunize-worlds-poorest-children.

Richter, J. (2004). Public-private Partnerships for health: A trend with no alternatives? Development, 47(2), 43–48. https://doi.org/10.1057/palgrave.development.1100043

Simon, C., & De Lemos, G. (2006). Unitaid: Un Financement innovant et solidaire pour lutter contre le Sida, le Paludisme et la Tuberculose. La Medicina Tropical, 2006(66), 583–584. https://www.jle.com/fr/MedSanteTrop/2006/66.6/583-584%20%20UNITAID%20un%20financement%20innovant%20et%20solidaire%20pour%20lutter%20contre%20le%20sida,%20le%20paludisme%20et%20la%20tuberculose%20(De%20L.pdf.

Syam, N. (2023). Leading and coordinating global health: Strengthening the World Health Organization, Research Paper No. 174. Geneva: South Centre, 13 February 2023. https://www.southcentre.int/research-paper-174-13-february-2023/.

Taylor, A. (2021). COVAX promised 2 billion doses of vaccine to help the world's poorest by 2021. It won't deliver even half that. The Washington Post, Dec 10, 2021. http://www.washingtonpost.com/world/2021/12/10/covax-doses-delivered/.

The Global Fund. (2025). History of the Global Fund. https://www.theglobalfund.org/en/about-the-global-fund/history-of-the-global-fund/.

United Nations. (2001a). United Nations General Assembly, 55th session, agenda item 173, A/RES/55/215, 6 March 2001. https://docs.un.org/en/%20A/RES/55/215.

United Nations. (2001b). United Nations General Assembly, 55th session, item 50 of the provisional agenda: Cooperation between the United Nations and all relevant partners, in particular the private sector, report by the Secretary General, 28 August 2001.

UN Global Compact. (2011). Secretary General of the United Nations, Ban Ki-moon. https://news.un.org/en/story/2011/06/379092-crucial-more-businesses-join-un-corporate-responsibility-pact-says-ban.

UN Global Compact. (2025). The ten principles of the UN global compact. https://unglobalcompact.org/what-is-gc/mission/principles.

UNICEF/UNDP/World Bank/WHO Special Programme for Research and Training in Tropical Diseases & World Health Organization. (2007). Making a difference : 30 years of research and capacity building for tropical diseases. World Health Organization. https://iris.who.int/handle/10665/43689.

Unitaid. (2017). L'impact de nos projets : Le Medicines Patent Pool. December 2017. https://unitaid.org/assets/L-impact-de-nos-projets-Medicines-Patent-Pool.pdf.

Unitaid. (2025). Unitaid website: About us. https://unitaid.org/about-unitaid/.

Vaughan, J. P., et al. (1996). Financing the World Health Organisation: global importance of extrabudgetary funds. Health Policy, 35(3), 229–245. https://doi.org/10.1016/0168-8510(95)00786-5. https://pubmed.ncbi.nlm.nih.gov/10157400/

Velásquez, G. (2014). Public-private partnerships in global health. Putting business before health? Research Paper No. 49. Geneva: South Centre, January 2014.

Velásquez, G. (2020). The World Health Organization reforms in the time of COVID-19, Research Paper No. 121. Geneva: South Centre, November 2020. https://www.southcentre.int/wp-content/uploads/2020/11/RP-121-rev2.pdf.

Velásquez, G. (2021). *Vacunas, medicamentos y patentes: COVID-19 y la necesidad de una Organización internacional*, 2021, Ed. B de F, Buenos Aires.

Velásquez, G. (2022). *Vaccines, medicines and COVID-19 how can be Given WHO a stronger voice?* SpringerBriefs in Public Health, (Springer & South Centre, 2022, Open Access). https://doi.org/10.1007/978-3-030-89125-1_1

WHO. (1998). Dr Gro Harlem Brundtland, Director-General Elect. Speech to the Fifty-first World Health Assembly Geneva, 13 May 1998Speech to the Fifty-first World Health Assembly. Geneva. A51/DIV/6, 13 May 1998. (pp. 4–5). https://apps.who.int/gb/archive/pdf_files/WHA51/eadiv6.pdf.

WHO. (2020). WHO Foundation Established to Support Critical Global Health Needs. Press Release, 27 May 2020, World Health Organization. https://www.who.int/news/item/27-05-2020-who-foundation-established-to-support-critical-global-health-needs

WHO. (2021). An appeal to G20 leaders to make vaccines accessible to people on the move Open letter to G20 Heads of State and Government, 29 October 2021. https://www.who.int/news/item/29-10-2021-an-appeal-to-g20-leaders-to-make-vaccines-accessible-to-people-on-the-move.

WHO. (2022). Meeting report of the working group on sustainable financing. EB/WGSF/7/4, 9 May 2022. https://apps.who.int/gb/wgsf/pdf_files/wgsf7/WGSF_7_4-en.pdf.

WHO (2025a). History of WHO. https://www.who.int/about/history.

WHO. (2025b). How WHO is funded. https://www.who.int/about/funding.

WHO. (2025c). A healthy return, Investment case for a sustainably financed WHO. https://www.who.int/about/funding/invest-in-who/investment-case-2.0.

WHO Foundation. (2020). Thomas Zeltner, Founder and Chairman of the WHO Foundation. https://who.foundation/.

World Bank. (2022). World Bank Board approves new fund for pandemic prevention, preparedness and response (PPR). Press Release, 30 June 2022. https://www.worldbank.org/en/news/press-release/2022/06/30/-world-bank-board-approves-new-fund-for-pandemic-prevention-preparedness-and-response-ppr.

World Bank and World Health Organization. (2017). Half the world lacks access to essential health services, 100 million people still tip into extreme poverty because of health spending. December 2017. https://www.who.int/news/item/13-12-2017-world-bank-and-who-half-the-world-lacks-access-to-essential-health-services-100-million-still-pushed-into-extreme-poverty-because-of-health-expenses

Chapter 4
WHO Negotiations on a Pandemic Treaty and the International Health Regulations Adopted in 2024

4.1 Introduction

The global response to the COVID-19 pandemic exposed numerous deficiencies. Several countries failed to adhere to WHO guidelines regarding preventive measures, quarantine protocols and standardized intensive care practices. Nonetheless, the most critical shortcoming was the inequitable distribution of diagnostics, vaccines and therapeutics. High-income nations amassed vaccine supplies far in excess of their actual needs, with large quantities ultimately expiring unused in storage facilities. This issue has received minimal scrutiny. Moreover, despite the fact that many of these medical innovations were developed with substantial public investment, their control was largely transferred to private industry.

The primary objective of the proposed pandemic treaty is to address the deficiencies exposed during the COVID-19 crisis and to establish a framework for more effective responses to future health emergencies. The pandemic underscored the critical need for coordinated and collective action, guided by the principles of public interest and global equity. However, as has become evident, these ideals were not realized in practice. In the meantime, the World Health Organization and scientific institutions continue to warn of the likely emergence of comparable global health threats.

Parts of this chapter are taken from: Velásquez, G. (2024 March 15). Where is the Binding International Treaty Negotiated at the WHO Against Future Pandemics Going? Southviews No. 259. https://www.southcentre.int/wp-content/uploads/2024/03/SV259_240315.pdf.

47

4.2   A Binding International Treaty Within the WHO

The proposal to create a legally binding international treaty within the framework of the WHO emerged after serious shortcomings became evident during the COVID-19 pandemic. The main issue was the unequal distribution and limited access to essential medical resources such as vaccines, diagnostics and treatments. This crisis clearly demonstrated the need for coordinated global action, guided by principles of equity, justice and public interest, although in practice these values were often ignored.

On 30 March 2021, in a moment of hope for building a fairer and more resilient world in the wake of COVID-19, 25 Heads of State, along with the President of the European Council, Charles Michel, and the WHO Director-General, Dr. Tedros Adhanom Ghebreyesus, advocated for the creation of an international pandemic treaty. Inspired by the lessons learned, this call led to the formal launch of negotiations in December 2021, resulting in the establishment of the Intergovernmental Negotiating Body (INB), with the mission of drafting an international instrument under the WHO focused on pandemic prevention, preparedness and response.

The final declaration of that meeting acknowledged that future pandemics are inevitable. It is not a question of if, but when. Therefore, the urgency of improving global preparedness through stronger prevention, detection, response and coordination mechanisms was emphasized. The need for a new international treaty centred on pandemic response was reaffirmed.

The health crisis between 2020 and 2023 revealed that the WHO lacks adequate legal tools or the necessary authority to enforce its recommendations and standards during health emergencies.

The scale of the global challenge posed by COVID-19 showed that no country can face a pandemic alone. Hence, the urgency to establish a binding international agreement that ensures equitable and timely access to medical resources in global health emergencies.

This treaty must be based on the principles of equity, inclusion and transparency, to guarantee fair and universal access to diagnostics, vaccines and treatments. Furthermore, it should be integrated into an international health system that strengthens the WHO's authority as the leading global health body. This would represent a significant shift in the approach to global health governance.

Thus, during its second special session in December 2021, the World Health Assembly formally created the INB, with the mandate to draft an international treaty in accordance with the WHO Constitution, under Article 19 or another deemed appropriate. This body operates under principles of consensus, member state leadership, efficiency, transparency and inclusion.

Additionally, the Assembly requested the WHO Director-General to support the INB's work by reporting on progress and organizing public hearings. Simultaneously, a process was initiated to review the International Health Regulations (2005), although the relationship between the two initiatives has not always been clear, generating confusion.

4.3 Treaty Negotiations: Progress, Tensions and Obstacles

Since its creation in December 2021, the Intergovernmental Negotiating Body (INB) has been working on the development of an international instrument to strengthen pandemic prevention, preparedness and response. However, the process has been marked by uneven progress, geopolitical tensions and significant differences among member states on key aspects of the agreement.

In the early rounds of negotiation, countries agreed on the need to improve global health response mechanisms. However, disagreements soon emerged on sensitive issues such as technology transfer, intellectual property, financing and especially equitable access to health products during crises.

One of the most debated points has been the creation of a system to ensure fair and rapid access to vaccines, medicines and diagnostics during future pandemics. Low- and middle-income countries have insisted that the treaty must establish firm commitments to prevent the recurrence of the inequalities seen during COVID-19. In contrast, several developed countries have been reluctant to accept provisions that might limit intellectual property rights or force them to share technologies without adequate compensation.

Another source of tension has been the proposal to establish a multilateral mechanism for sharing information on pathogens with pandemic potential, as well as the benefits derived from their use. This system, based on the principle of reciprocity, seeks to ensure that countries providing biological resources also receive fair benefits if derived products are developed. However, its implementation has raised doubts about its legal, technical and political feasibility.

The INB has also faced challenges regarding the role the WHO should play in coordinating and overseeing the treaty. While some states support a stronger role for the WHO, others prefer to maintain national sovereignty as the central pillar of health response. This has complicated the definition of compliance and monitoring mechanisms to ensure that treaty provisions are respected by all signatories.

Despite these obstacles, the INB has made progress in drafting a consolidated text, with multiple versions and comments reflecting divergent positions. This process has been accompanied by regional consultations, public hearings and the participation of non-state actors, including civil society organizations, academic experts and private sector representatives.

The initial goal was to adopt the treaty during the 77th World Health Assembly in May 2024. However, due to the complexity of the negotiations and the lack of consensus on key issues, this objective was not achieved. It is now considered likely that the process will extend beyond 2024, raising doubts about the real political will to advance towards a fairer and more solidarity-based global health governance.

In summary, although the negotiation process has allowed significant progress in the discussion on international health governance, there is still a long way to go to achieve a truly transformative agreement. The success of the treaty will depend on the member states' ability to overcome their differences and prioritize the common interest above national or corporate interests.

4.4   Country Positions: Interests, Tensions and Alliances

The negotiation process of the pandemic treaty has revealed deep asymmetries among countries, not only in their technical and financial capacities but also in their political and strategic priorities. These differences have resulted in a complex web of alliances, tensions and disputes that reflect both the structural inequalities of the international system and the lessons (and resentments) from the management of the COVID-19 pandemic.

Low- and middle-income countries, especially those from the Global South, have consistently advocated for a treaty that ensures equitable access to essential health products during health emergencies. These nations have demanded the inclusion of binding mechanisms for technology transfer, intellectual property flexibility, sustained pandemic preparedness financing and a fairer model for distributing vaccines, diagnostics and treatments.

These demands have been supported by blocs such as the African Group, the Latin American and Caribbean Group (GRULAC) and the Alliance of Least Developed Countries, which have sought to consolidate common positions to strengthen their negotiating power against high-income countries.

On the other hand, several Global North states—including the United States, the European Union and its member states, the United Kingdom, Switzerland and Japan—have taken more conservative stances. While they recognize the importance of improving global pandemic response, they have emphasized the need to preserve innovation incentives, protect intellectual property rights and avoid commitments that could affect the competitiveness of their pharmaceutical industries.

These countries have also insisted that international cooperation should be based on the principles of voluntariness, sovereignty and respect for national regulatory frameworks. As a result, they have rejected proposals involving strict legal obligations or robust compliance mechanisms, especially regarding equitable access and benefit-sharing.

In this context, some strategic alliances have gained strength. The Group of 77 plus China, for example, has been a key actor in advocating for a transformative and equity-centred treaty. In contrast, the so-called "Friends of the Treaty" group—mainly composed of high-income countries—has promoted a more technical, limited approach aimed at capacity-building without altering the status quo in global health trade and innovation.

Likewise, non-state actors such as civil society organizations, academic networks and international cooperation agencies have sought to influence the negotiations, either by supporting Global South demands or by denouncing the resistance of the Global North to introduce substantive reforms to the global health regime.

In summary, the negotiation process for the pandemic treaty reflects not only a technical debate over preparedness and response models, but also a deeper struggle over the kind of health governance we aim to build: one centred on equity and international solidarity, or one that perpetuates the dominant logics of market forces and national sovereignty.

4.5   The Failure of Negotiations on a Binding Treaty to Prevent Future Pandemics

A small group of industrialized countries, including the major pharmaceutical industry, opposed the text of the binding treaty to prevent future pandemics that had been under negotiation at the WHO for 2 years. These countries chose to protect the private interests of their pharmaceutical industry. The countries of the South, despite having a large majority, were unable to push through a text based on the general interest, in defence of the health of all the world's citizens. Once again, private commercial interests have been placed above the public interest under the impotent eyes of the WHO Secretariat and without heeding the critical appeals of experts, organizations such as the South Centre, health NGOs and academic observers following the dossier.

On 10 May 2024, the WHO issued a Press Release titled "Governments agree to continue their steady progress on proposed pandemic agreement ahead of the World Health Assembly" (WHO, 2024). It sounds like a self-proclaimed victory—what an understatement! The WHO member countries did not agree on anything, they simply acknowledged that the two-year negotiation—which was the deadline set by all the member countries to define the treaty—had failed. The intergovernmental negotiating body tasked with drafting a document to be presented for adoption at the World Health Assembly in June 2024, on the last day of its mandate, was no longer working on the text but on how to renew its mandate...

If the negotiations are to continue, the first thing to do would be to analyse, identify and acknowledge the reasons why the negotiations failed within the planned timeframe.

The three most debated points are as follows:

1. That of the barriers that intellectual property and the use of patents can pose during a pandemic (article 11 of the draft document, which was not adopted).
2. The Pathogen Access and Benefit-Sharing System (PABS). This system means that the provision of information on a pathogen—essential for the development of vaccines and treatments—would be linked to a mechanism guaranteeing access to health products developed on the basis of this data. According to the latest version of the failed draft treaty, the WHO would reserve 20 percent of the global production of medicines produced under the PABS—half free of charge, the other half at a preferential price—for developing countries (article 12 of the aborted draft).
3. The "One Health" concept. The EU has put pressure on developing countries to accept the proposal to develop a legally binding instrument on the "One Health" approach. It should be noted that there is no mandate in the INB and no consensus to negotiate a stand-alone instrument on the "One Health" approach. The development of an instrument covering all aspects of the "One Health" approach will require addressing issues that go beyond the scope of the pandemic treaty being negotiated in the WHO.

The draft text of Article 5 of the INB reads as follows: "The Parties, recognising that most emerging infectious diseases and pandemics are caused by zoonotic pathogens, commit themselves, in the context of pandemic prevention, preparedness, response and recovery of health systems, to promote and implement the 'One Health' approach, at national and, where appropriate, regional and global levels, which is coherent, integrated, coordinated and concerted among all relevant actors, applying national legislation and existing instruments and initiatives".

The first problem that makes it difficult to deal with these three problematic points (and other points in the document on which there was no agreement) stems from what might be considered a dual, even schizophrenic, position in the major declarations by the Heads of States[1] of the industrialized countries (WHO, 2020). On the one hand, they claim to consider medicines as global public goods, but on the other, they defend and try to impose the opposite, i.e., that medicines are health products, as can be seen in the discussions with the negotiators from these countries (as was the case in the negotiation of the INB in 2021–2024).

The second problem with the negotiations, and probably the most serious, is the abandonment of the concept of essential medicines (which covers vaccines, diagnostics and treatments) developed over 40 years by the WHO and adopted by the vast majority of developing countries. It has been replaced by the ambiguous term *health or medical countermeasures*", a term that means nothing in terms of public health but alludes to security and the wars to be contained (O'Neill Institute, Foundation for the National Institutes of Health and University of Cape Town, 2023). In reality, "medical countermeasures" refer to health products, which the major pharmaceutical industries in industrialized countries use as commercial weapons, and not to essential medicines, which can be considered as public goods.

The third general problem with the text that was not adopted is that it marks a clear step backwards on the issue of intellectual property rights compared with the texts adopted 17 years ago at the WHO (WHO, 2008). We can see from the wording of the text that we are moving from the *mandatory use of TRIPS flexibilities* to the ambiguous language of "*mutually agreed voluntary measures*".

The developed countries have significantly diluted the original draft, introducing numerous unwarranted qualifications. Phrases such as "where appropriate" and other language characteristic of non-binding provisions are repeated throughout the text.

It is not a question of continuing negotiations to "refine the current draft", as the WHO press release puts it. The document needs to be substantially redrafted so that it contains legally binding measures that address the problem of access to the R&D and technologies needed to produce essential medicines for future pandemics.

The current draft text of the binding treaty to prevent future pandemics, which must be the subject of new negotiations, falls far short of responding adequately to the challenges raised during the COVID-19 crisis.

---

[1] More than 10 heads of state addressed the World Health Assembly in May 2020 to argue that future medicines, vaccines and treatments for COVID-19 should be considered global public goods.

4.6   The New International Health Regulations

The amendments to the International Health Regulations (IHR) approved at the 77th World Health Assembly (in June 2024) do not represent a substantial step forward in preparing the world for health crises similar to that of COVID-19.

"The amendments have been hailed as a victory for multilateralism and global health. The amendments identified as the most significant, however, do not constitute game-changing reforms, especially concerning low-income countries' demands for equity and financial assistance, on which the negotiations reached, at best, a truce" (Fidler, 2024).

General references to equity and solidarity do not translate into operational mechanisms to ensure equitable access, such as those mentioned in Article 13(9)(b) and (c):

> (b) engaging with and encouraging relevant stakeholders operating in their respective jurisdictions to facilitate equitable access to relevant health products in response to a public health emergency of international concern, including a pandemic emergency; and
>
> (c) make available, where appropriate, the relevant terms of its research and development agreements for the medical devices concerned, with a view to promoting equitable access to such devices during a public health emergency of international concern, including a pandemic emergency.

Other changes, such as the power to declare a pandemic emergency, do nothing to solve the problems caused by COVID-19 and do nothing to prevent the adoption by many industrialized countries of what has been called vaccine nationalism.

One of the main revisions of the IHR in 2005 was the granting to the WHO Director-General of the power to declare a public health emergency of international concern (PHEIC), despite the objections of the countries directly affected. The declaration of a public health emergency of international concern applies to events that have the potential to become pandemics.

The amendments to IHR 2024 formalize the obvious, namely that a pandemic emergency is a specific type of PHEIC, and therefore establish that the WHO Director-General can declare a pandemic emergency. COVID-19 was a PHEIC that the WHO Director-General declared a pandemic. This clarification in no way changes the way the IHR operate. A pandemic emergency is a PHEIC, and no one has questioned the fact that the concept of PHEIC encompasses diseases that were pandemics.

The amendments to the IHR did not adopt a progressive approach to the different levels of PHEIC required by certain countries.

Another change considered important is the requirement for parties to the IHR to designate a national authority responsible for coordinating implementation of the IHR. The IHR 2005 already required parties to have an IHR National Focal Point responsible for national implementation.

4.7   Reference to Financing

The IHR 2005 did not require developed countries to provide financial assistance to help developing countries meet their IHR obligations. Nor does it refer to financing.

References to how the implementation of the IHR will be funded are made in Article 44 "Collaboration, assistance and funding" and Article 44a "Coordination".

It could be argued that progress has been made insofar as the new IHR 2024 makes reference to funding, which the IHR 2005 did not do. However, the references to Articles 44 and 44a are vague and unclear, with paragraphs such as:

> (b) seek to maximize the availability of funds to meet the implementation needs and priorities of States Parties, in particular developing countries; and
> (c) endeavour to mobilize new and additional financial resources and to increase the efficiency of the use of existing funding instruments, with a view to the effective implementation of this Regulation.

These references are far from constituting a concrete and sustainable funding mechanism that countries can call on in the event of a pandemic. Point 3 of Article 44a, which some see as an unfinished solution, reads as follows: "3. the mechanism shall, in respect of the implementation of this Regulation, operate under the authority and direction of the Health Assembly and be accountable to it". This sentence is nothing more than a vague hope that if, in the end, there is no funding for the implementation of the IHR, countries will be able to start "knocking on the door" of the WHA again.

During COVID-19, developing countries noted the lack of financial assistance for access to vaccines and health products and denounced the lack of equity and collective action on this issue, as COVAX took place outside the IHR.

The amendments on the means of financing in the new IHR 2024 are weak, with vague obligations such as "promoting the identification of funding sources and mobilising voluntary contributions for this implementation" and are subject to "applicable legislation and available resources".

4.8   Creation of a Committee of States Parties

Finally, the changes in the IHR 2024 have incorporated the idea of creating a Committee of States Parties, which will meet every 2 years to facilitate implementation. The Committee is not a compliance and accountability mechanism. Its mandate is "to *be solely facilitative and consultative in nature, and to operate in a non-confrontational, non-punitive, supportive and transparent manner*" and to promote and support "*learning, exchange of good practices and cooperation*". This committee does not represent a significant change; in all previous health crises, the WHA has requested evaluations of the management of these crises.

4.9 "Progress" for the United States

The United States led and accepted the 2005 revision as well as the recent 2024 revision.

The outcome of the negotiations on the amendments is mainly in the interests of the United States. Amendments have been accepted that do not alter the operation of the IHR and do not impose substantial binding obligations on the IHR in terms of equity and financial assistance. The "new" provisions on equity, funding and regular meetings of the parties to the IHR 2024 do not substantially change the situation in the event of future pandemics.

The urgency of the United States and the European Union to approve the IHR at the WHA 2024, while leaving the negotiations on a pandemic treaty open, was no doubt due to the desire of the industrialized countries that the negotiations on the pandemic treaty should not "contaminate" the IHR on issues such as access to vaccines, medicines and diagnostic tools.

References

Fidler, D. P. (2024). The amendments to the international health regulations are not a breakthrough. ThinkGlobalHealth, 7 June 2024. https://www.thinkglobalhealth.org/article/amendments-international-health-regulations-are-not-breakthrough.

O'Neill Institute, Foundation for the National Institutes of Health and University of Cape Town. (2023). Emergency countermeasure development and deployment. Global pandemic agreement: WHO collaborating center support for new equity and coordinating mechanisms. November 2023. https://fnih.org/wp-content/uploads/2023/11/Emergency-Countermeasure-Development-and-Deployment-1-November-2023.pdf.

WHO. (2008). Global strategy and plan of action on public health, innovation and intellectual property. WHA61.21, 24 May 2008. https://apps.who.int/gb/ebwha/pdf_files/a61/a61_r21-en.pdf.

WHO. (2020). Global leaders unite to ensure everyone everywhere can access new vaccines, tests and treatments for COVID-19. Press release, 24 April 2020. https://www.who.int/news/item/24-04-2020-global-leaders-unite-to-ensure-everyone-everywhere-can-access-new-vaccines-tests-and-treatments-for-covid-19.

WHO. (2024). Governments agree to continue their steady progress on proposed pandemic agreement ahead of the World Health Assembly. Press Release 10 May 2024. https://www.who.int/news/item/10-05-2024-governments-agree-to-continue-their-steady-progress-on-proposed-pandemic-agreement-ahead-of-the-world-health-assembly

Chapter 5
Building a Latin American and Caribbean Medicines Agency

5.1 Introduction

The "Acapulco Declaration" for the establishment of the Latin American and Caribbean Medicines and Medical Devices Regulatory Agency (AMLAC, which stands for "Agencia latinoamericana y del caribe de medicamentos") was signed by the drug regulatory bodies of Colombia (INVIMA), Cuba (CECMED) and Mexico (COFEPRIS) on April 26, 2023, in Acapulco, Mexico (INVIMA-CECMED-COFEPRIS, 2023).

Through the harmonization and convergence of health standards and the establishment of a regional medicines market in Latin America, AMLAC was established to support regional integration and guarantee access to high-quality, safe and effective medications and medical devices. This chapter looks at the background, standards and goals behind the establishment of AMLAC.

The "Acapulco Declaration" proposed the establishment of AMLAC as a mechanism to advance regional integration by promoting the harmonization and convergence of health regulations. Its primary objective is to ensure equitable access to safe, effective and high-quality medicines and medical devices. Furthermore, the Declaration extended an invitation to the national regulatory authorities of Argentina, Brazil and Chile to participate in this initiative. It also called upon the South Centre—an intergovernmental organization representing developing countries, including Colombia, Cuba and others in the region—to offer both technical and political support at the international level.

In addition, it was agreed that the Pro Tempore Presidency of the Community of Latin American and Caribbean States (PPT-CELAC) would be regularly informed

This chapter is largely taken from: Velásquez, G. (2023 July 11). Towards A Latin American and Caribbean Medicines Agency (AMLAC). South Centre Policy Brief No. 120. https://www.south-centre.int/wp-content/uploads/2023/07/PB120_Towards-A-Latin-American-and-Caribbean-Medicines-Agency_EN.pdf. Used with permission.

57

about the development of AMLAC. This measure is intended to foster broad knowledge exchange and encourage input from interested member states.

The leaders of the drug regulatory agencies in Argentina, Brazil, Chile, Colombia, Cuba and Mexico convened in Bogotá, Colombia, from 15–17 June 2023, and decided to gradually establish a drug agency for Latin America and the Caribbean.

This proposal aligns with the Declaration issued by the Ministers of Health of the Community of Latin American and Caribbean States (CELAC) on 24 November 2022, which affirms: "Confirm that medicines, vaccines, treatments and other health technologies developed in response to a public health emergency are global public goods and an essential element of the right to health. (...) Maintain a strong commitment to any regional or global initiative aimed at facilitating universal and equitable access to medicines, vaccines, treatments and other health technologies (...)" (CELAC, 2022).

5.2 General Context

As part of its constitutional mandate, the World Health Organization (WHO) is tasked with "developing, establishing, and promoting international standards concerning food, biological, pharmaceutical, and similar products" (WHO, 1946). In line with this responsibility, the WHO has actively worked over the past three decades to support and encourage countries in formulating pharmaceutical policies as integral components of their national health strategies. Additionally, the Organization has played a key role in establishing technical standards—such as Good Manufacturing Practices—through its expert committees. However, the regulation of medicines remains a sovereign responsibility, with individual States bearing the obligation to establish their own national medicines regulatory authorities.

The primary regulatory bodies in industrialized nations including France,[1] the UK, Germany, Spain, Australia, Japan and Canada were established just 30 to 40 years ago, with the exception of the US Food and Drug Administration (FDA), which was established in 1906.

Over the past 30 years, several drug regulatory organizations have been established throughout Latin America, including COFEPRIS in Mexico in 2001, ANAMED in Chile in 2016, INVIMA in Colombia in 1994, ANVISA in Brazil in 1999, ANMAT in Argentina in 1992 and CECMED in Cuba in 1989. These agencies are classified as level IV by the WHO.

The primary aim of these regulatory agencies is to safeguard public health by overseeing and ensuring the quality, safety and effectiveness of medicines and medical devices.

---

[1] *L'Agence nationale de sécurité du médicament et des produits de santé* (ANSM). https://ansm.sante.fr/.

In 1980, the World Health Organization (WHO) established the International Conference of Drug Regulatory Authorities (ICDRA), which convenes biennially. Subsequently, in 1999, the Pan American Health Organization (PAHO) initiated the Pan-American Conference on Drug Regulation. Unlike the WHO ICDRA, this forum includes participation from the pharmaceutical industry, which also contributes to its financing.

The European Medicines Agency (EMA) is a European Union agency set up in 1995. Since 2019, it has been based in Amsterdam. With the United Kingdom's exit from the European Union, the agency moved from London to the Netherlands.

In February 2019, the States of the African Union signed a treaty establishing the African Medicines Agency (African Union, 2019).

5.3   The International Council for Harmonization of Technical Requirements for Pharmaceuticals for Human Use

In April 1990, representatives of European, Japanese and American pharmaceutical industry associations and regulatory bodies created the International Council for Harmonization of Technical Requirements for Pharmaceuticals for Human Use (ICH), formerly known as the International Conference on Harmonization.

Since the establishment of the International Council for Harmonization (ICH) in 1990, the World Health Organization (WHO) has shown hesitation in joining an initiative on international health regulations that was initiated, promoted and funded by the pharmaceutical industries of the United States, the European Union and Japan. Following complex internal debates,[2] the WHO chose to participate with an ambiguous "observer" status, a position it has maintained for over three decades.

At the World Health Assembly in May 2015, the United States and the European Union introduced a draft resolution calling on WHO Member States to adopt ICH standards for pharmaceuticals. However, this proposal was ultimately rejected due to opposition led by Argentina and Colombia on behalf of developing countries.

Although the 2015 World Health Assembly successfully stopped the adoption of commercially driven standards in place of public health-oriented ones, the International Council for Harmonization (ICH) continues to function alongside the regulatory authorities of industrialized nations, the European Medicines Agency and even the WHO. The ICH has fostered a regulatory culture that continues to influence national drug authorities. However, the issue extends beyond the ICH itself—it reflects the broader structure and underlying philosophy of

---

[2] In 1990, the WHO had two departments responsible for pharmaceutical products, with different policies and strategies. One department was very close to the European and American pharmaceutical industry, while the other, where the author was based, was closer to developing countries, and defended clearer public health principles and standards for medicines clearly based on public health rather than the commercial interests of the pharmaceutical industry.

pharmaceutical research and development in industrialized countries, where the sector operates primarily as a business enterprise rather than a public health service. This commercial orientation has proven to be highly lucrative, as evidenced by the rapid development and global marketing of COVID-19 vaccines over the past 2 years.

In today's globalized world, it is imperative that pharmaceutical regulatory standards and practices be harmonized. Determining the standards and goals of this kind of harmonization represents a challenge.

The ICH seeks to harmonize pharmaceutical regulations, with its principal aim being the protection of the markets of the companies that finance its operations. National regulatory agencies operate under two often conflicting pressures: on one hand, the commercial interests of the pharmaceutical industry, and on the other, the responsibility of the State to safeguard public health by ensuring the quality, safety and efficacy of medicines.

The ICH adopts stringent standards that often do not align with genuine public health needs but instead function to marginalize pharmaceutical industries in developing countries, effectively limiting competition.

It is widely acknowledged that many ICH-endorsed regulations are designed more to safeguard commercial markets than to protect patient welfare. Under the guise of harmonizing regulatory requirements for drug approvals, regulatory authorities from high-income countries—alongside three major pharmaceutical industry associations—have used the ICH framework, established in 1990, to advance their own interests by imposing their evaluation criteria globally. At times, the ICH's recommended toxicity standards prioritize quicker and more cost-effective drug development over patient safety, while its quality requirements can raise production costs without delivering clear health benefits. Ideally, the World Health Organization should assume leadership in establishing drug development standards, ensuring they prioritize patient needs above market considerations (Prescrire International, 2010).

As part of the ICH-promoted "culture", health registration has evolved into a complicated, time-consuming and laborious marketing authorization process. Its commercial worth comes from the fact that it is the "gateway" to the market.

Health registrations are regarded as intangible "assets" because, in a sense, the holder of a registration has "passed" a series of tests that aren't always transparent, objective or defined in terms of the actual "stakeholders" of the regulatory bodies, which aren't pharmaceutical companies but rather society at large.

A result of this "culture" is the excessive quantity of medications in use in the majority of countries. For instance, the World Health Organization reports that 7500 medications are permitted for distribution in Switzerland, 12,000 in South Africa, 13,500 in the Netherlands, 17,000 in Colombia and 56,000 in Argentina. There are, however, just 479 medicines in the 2021 revision of the WHO Model List of Essential Medicines.

The administrative procedure of registration has essentially replaced health monitoring. Good manufacturing practices (GMPs) and producer operating licences are valuable, but what matters most are the registrations. Furthermore, when it comes to issuing sanitary registrations, developing countries undertake a lot more paperwork analysis than on-site monitoring.

5.4   Suggested Principles and Goals for a Latin American Food and Drug Regulatory Agency

There is a pressing need to establish an autonomous regulatory body guided primarily by public health priorities and tailored to the region's social, economic, industrial and healthcare realities.

- Develop and implement regulations and standards to ensure the quality, safety and efficacy of medicines and related health products, strictly based on public health needs.
- Streamline and harmonize market authorization requirements to support the growth of a regional pharmaceutical sector and facilitate a unified Latin American market for medicines and medical devices.
- Prevent the adoption of technical standards that are misaligned with regional health priorities and could hinder the development of domestic pharmaceutical industries.
- The agency could improve the health registration process. For instance, Nordic countries once refused to approve drugs offering no added value over existing treatments. In contrast, many regional agencies currently approve marginal or inferior products, often driven by aggressive marketing rather than therapeutic merit.
- A regional authority could also reduce redundancy in regulatory processes. Procedures and requirements should be harmonized using criteria that reflect the region's health priorities, support industrial development and suit the economic conditions of Latin American nations.
- Create a regional medicines registry aligned with WHO guidelines for essential medicine selection.
- Encourage broader acceptance and use of generic medicines.
- Set standards for approving biological products and biosimilars (generic versions of biologics).
- Coordinate with national patent offices to align medicine patenting practices with public health goals.
- Design a funding model that does not rely solely on registration fees from pharmaceutical companies. Such dependence may incentivize an excessive number of approvals, potentially at the expense of public health interests.

5.5   Concluding Remarks

In the United States, the European Union and Japan, the research, production and marketing of pharmaceuticals are extremely lucrative sectors where commerce and financial gain are prioritized over the welfare and health of the population. In contrast, countries like Colombia, Cuba and Mexico (through the Acapulco Declaration), along with Argentina, Brazil, Chile, Colombia, Cuba and Mexico (in the Bogotá Meeting on Regulatory Convergence), are now striving to establish a Latin American medicines agency that places health at the forefront. Their goal is to treat medicines not merely as commercial products but as public goods that serve to protect and restore people's health. With a regional market of 500 million people, positioning medicines as public goods could also bring significant economic benefits to Latin America.

References

African Union. (2019). Treaty for the Establishment of the African Medicines Agency (AMA). https://au.int/en/treaties/treaty-establishment-african-medicines-agency.

CELAC. (2022). Declaration of the Ministers of Health of the Community of Latin American and Caribbean States (CELAC) of 24 November 2022.

INVIMA-CECMED-COFEPRIS. (2023). Acapulco Declaration, 26 April 2023. https://www.cecmed.cu/noticias/declaracion-acapulco-creacion-agencia-reguladora-medicamentos-dispositivos-medicos.

Prescrire International. (2010). ICH: An exclusive club of drug regulatory agencies and drug companies imposing its rules on the rest of the world. *Prescrire International, 19*(108), 183–186.

WHO. (1946). WHO Constitution, Article 2 (u). https://apps.who.int/gb/bd/pdf/bd47/en/constitution-en.pdf.

Chapter 6
From the Concept of "Essential Medicines" to That of "Medical Countermeasures"

6.1 Introduction

One example of how international health negotiations can weaken and undermine fundamental public health concepts developed by the WHO and many WHO member countries is the concept of *"essential medicines"*, which has been replaced by the term *"medical countermeasures" or "health countermeasures"*.

The concept of "essential medicines" launched by the WHO in 1977 in response to the proliferation of pharmaceutical products on the markets of many countries is undoubtedly one of the major successes of this organization in its history. The debate on access to diagnostics, vaccines and treatments had been included in the concept of essential medicines for 50 years.

In the crisis provoked by the COVID-19 pandemic, many of us believed that it would lead us to rethink a better world, but paradoxically, in certain areas, it represented a step backwards. Some have developed ambiguous terms with little public health content, such as "medical countermeasures" or "health countermeasures". These "new" terms are closer to "health products" than to common public goods.[1]

6.2 The Concept of Essential Medicines

The industrial manufacture of medicines was not yet 100 years old. With the appearance of sulphonamides (1935), antibiotics (1944) and anti-tuberculosis drugs (1945), there was talk of a "therapeutic revolution" and "miracle drugs". These drugs made it possible to treat diseases that had previously been fatal, giving the

---

[1] During the COVID-19 pandemic, at the 2020 World Health Assembly, more than 10 heads of state described future vaccines as public goods.

© The Author(s), under exclusive license to Springer Nature Switzerland AG 2025
G. Velásquez, *Negotiating Global Health Policies*, SpringerBriefs in Public Health, https://doi.org/10.1007/978-3-031-99847-8_6

pharmaceutical industry the prestige it enjoyed until the end of the 1990s (Velásquez, 1991).

Between 1985 and 2000, the number of new molecules accepted, for example by the FDA, fell by three quarters (Even & Debré, 2012). From the early 2000s to the present day, we have witnessed the advent of biological drugs that completely decouple R&D and production costs from sales prices. "Biological drugs represent only 2 percent of drugs on the market, but 37 percent of total pharmaceutical expenditure in the United States" (ACMA, 2023).

Here are a few examples of these "new" drugs that are highly effective but not accessible to everyone who needs them: Sofosbuvir (2014) for hepatitis C, from the US company Gilead, costing $84,000 for a three-month course of treatment. Orkambi (2015) for fibrosis in 2-year-olds, from the US firm Vertex, 133,000 US dollars per dose. Kymriah (2018) for leukaemia, from the Swiss company Novartis, 320,000 euros; Zolgensma (2019) for muscular atrophy in newborns, from the Swiss company Novartis, 2,100,000 US dollars per dose (Swissinfo, 2019; Annett, 2021); Hemgenix "Haemophilia Gene Therapy" (2023), the most expensive drug in the history of the pharmaceutical industry, a single-dose treatment costing 3.5 million US dollars, from the American company CSL Behring (Naddaf and Nature Magazine, 2022).

The debate on essential medicines arose after the boom in the industrial development of the pharmaceutical industry. Between 1950 and 1960, for example, 3800 new products were introduced onto the US market, and between 1960 and 1970, the rate of new products entering the market accelerated still further.

Faced with this proliferation of products on the market, which posed multiple problems of quality control and access, and taking into account the inspiring experience of certain countries, such as Peru and Sri Lanka, which had adopted the "basic medicines" or "essential medicines" approach to improve their population's access to adequate medicines, the WHO set up a committee of experts in 1977 to answer the following question: how many medicines are really needed to meet the needs of the population? After concluding that some 220 medicines could be considered essential for the proper practice of medicine, the Committee drew up a model list.

6.3   The Model List of Essential Medicines

Essential medicines are those that satisfy the priority health care needs of a population. They are selected with due regard to disease prevalence and public health relevance, evidence of efficacy and safety and comparative cost-effectiveness. They are intended to be available in functioning health systems at all times, in appropriate dosage forms, of assured quality and at prices individuals and health systems can afford (WHO, 2023a).

The first model list of essential medicines, published in 1977 by the WHO, triggered a major international controversy in the health sector. Indignation, surprise, hostility from the medical profession and even resistance from the pharmaceutical industry. The *Syndicat national de l'Industrie pharmaceutique française*, for example, reacted very strongly to the publication of the list of essential medicines, in a letter to the newspaper Le Monde: "In the name of what principle can an organization, even an international one, advise limiting existing weapons in the fight against disease, knowing that part of the population is at risk, knowing that part of the population will be deprived of care corresponding to its needs?" (Le Monde, 1979).

Today, 40 years later, in both developed and developing countries, no one in the scientific or academic circles seriously questions the principle of the list of essential medicines recommended by the WHO. This list has been revised every 2 years since 1977. The current version, updated in July 2023, is the 23rd list of essential medicines (WHO, 2023b).

> Today, essential medicines are linked to public goods, human rights and a public health revolution based on primary health care. However, for hundreds of millions of people, the enjoyment of this public good, the enjoyment of this human right and participation in this health revolution are out of reach. This publication is therefore the story of a challenge, but also of an unfinished story.....[2]

The principle of selecting and limiting medicines is neither new, nor a feature of "second-rate medicine for underdeveloped countries". Long before this recommendation was proclaimed by the WHO, this measure was practised by the best-known hospitals in the United States, Sweden, the Netherlands, Switzerland and elsewhere. Hospitals in these countries work with lists of 300 to 500 medicines, which demonstrates the economic and therapeutic rationality of this measure.

The changes recommended at the last review of the essential medicines list in 2023 bring the total number of medicines (including fixed-dose combinations) on the essential medicines list to 502 products (from 479 in 2021) (WHO, 2023b).

"Because of the great differences between countries, the preparation of a drug list of uniform, general applicability is not feasible or possible" (WHO, 1990). It is therefore up to each country to adapt the WHO Model List of Essential Medicines to its own economic and social situation and health policies. The WHO list is a model that countries can use to determine their own priorities and choices. However, the main criteria for selecting products for a national essential medicines list are as follows:

- therapeutic needs in relation to the diseases prevalent in the country
- the efficacy, safety and quality of medicines
- the diagnostic and treatment resources available in the country
- the training and experience of the staff available
- the financial resources available and the cost of drugs
- medicines containing a single active substance (with a few rare exceptions).

---

[2] Foreword by Halfdan Mahler, former Director of the WHO, in the book by F. Antezana and X. Seuba. Seuba "Medicamentos esenciales, historia de un desafío" ed. ICARIA, Barcelona, 2008.

6.4 Action Programme on Essential Medicines

The establishment of a national list does not necessarily lead to the implementation of the list or the concept of essential medicines. In some countries, the new list remains a paper exercise. Many countries continue to import and use non-essential, expensive and unnecessary medicines. To resolve the problems posed by the purchase and use of medicines, the list of essential medicines needed to be part of a pharmaceutical policy, itself a component of a national health policy. In 1981, the WHO set up the Action Programme on Essential Medicines. The Action Programme on Essential Medicines was created as an operational programme to help countries develop national medicines policies.

> The objective of the Action Programme on Essential Medicines is to work with countries to ensure the regular supply, at the lowest possible cost, and rational use of a defined number of medicines and vaccines of acceptable quality, safety and efficacy (WHO Division of Drug Management and Policies, 1988).

To achieve this objective, the programme helps countries to develop and implement national pharmaceutical policies based on the concept of essential medicines and primary healthcare policy.

6.5 Components of a National Pharmaceutical Policy

The components of a national pharmaceutical policy can be grouped under eight main headings:

- Drug selection: identification of therapeutic needs; quantification; information; utilization studies.
- Drug supply: procurement, manufacturing, local formulation, distribution, logistics.
- Rational use of medicines: training and information on medicines for human use.
- Doctors, pharmacists, other health specialists and the general public.
- Quality assurance: of medicines produced, bought and sold.
- Legislation and regulations: laws and regulations, supervisory authorities.
- Financial resources: analysis of financial needs, financing methods.
- Technology transfer and development, pharmaceutical research and development.
- Developing the potential of local knowledge and therapeutic resources.
- Strategies for managing intellectual property in the pharmaceutical sector from a public health perspective.

6.6 Current Situation and Outlook

Access to essential medicines remains very critical, for reasons such as scarcity of resources, inadequate infrastructure and lack of technical and managerial staff, particularly in developing countries. These problems have been exacerbated in recent years, notably during the COVID-19 pandemic, by the widespread use of patents in developing countries following the creation of the World Trade Organization (WTO) in 1995 and the adoption of the TRIPS Agreement.

The relationship between the public and private sectors remains a key factor in achieving the objectives of the essential medicines policy, a factor that is not clear to the WHO and which has still not been resolved.

In 2002, in an article published celebrating 25 years of the "essential medicines" concept, the authors stated: "For newer medicines, the World Trade Organization (WTO) Agreement on Trade-Related Aspects of Intellectual Property Rights (TRIPS) has established for WTO members a global minimum for patent protection. Many experts predict that, unless countries appropriately apply TRIPS safeguards and unless further progress is made to deal with some of the outstanding issues concerning the TRIPS agreement, the price of new drugs will be unaffordable for many millions of people" (Quick et al., 2002).

6.7 Where Does the Expression "Medical Countermeasures" or "Health Countermeasures" Come From?

The O'Neill Institute at Georgetown University in Washington is a WHO Collaborating Centre, which organized a meeting of experts in November 2023[3] to "support the work of the World Health Assembly (WHA) and the Intergovernmental Negotiating Body for a future treaty on pandemics" (INB). This meeting, which followed "Chatham House rules",[4] resulted in the publication of a document which summarized the discussions, elaborated and introduced the term "technical or health countermeasures" to support the work of the WHA and the INB. "This report summarises the main themes that emerged during the meeting, for use by policy makers and the international community in considering how to move forward" (O'Neill Institute, Foundation for the National Institutes of Health, University of Cape Town, 2023).

---

[3] Experts "representing" all WHO regions in disciplines as diverse as global health, law, human rights, biomedical science, financial services, civil society, intellectual property, the life sciences industry, clinical trial design, government, retail health, patient advocacy, the environment, academia and health equity", the document states.

[4] Under the "Chatham House Rule", anyone taking part in a meeting is free to use information from the debate, but cannot reveal who made a particular comment. This rule is a system for organising debates and round tables on controversial issues. It takes its name from the London headquarters of the Royal Institute of International Affairs, where it was founded in June 1927.

The summary report states that *"This summary report is not meant as a consensus document,* but as a compilation of the ideas and diverse perspectives offered by experts who are participating in their individual capacity, not as representatives of their respective organisations. Presenting the landscape of views is intentional and no expert is expected to endorse every single point contained in the report. In fact, it is likely that every expert will disagree with various assertions incorporated herein. Moreover, language included in this document does not imply institutional endorsement by the organisations that participants represent" (O'Neill Institute, Foundation for the National Institutes of Health, and University of Cape Town 2023). Despite this cautious preamble, the report makes it clear from the introduction that the *emergency countermeasures are vaccines, diagnostics and treatments.*

In an article published in Lancet authored by Roland Alexander Driece, Precious Matsoso et al. (co-chairs of the INB and participants in the O'Neil Institute meeting under Chatham House rules), the term *"countermeasures"* is introduced to refer to vaccines, drugs and diagnostics (Driece, Matsoso et al. 2023).

The conclusions of the O'Neil Institute's report clearly state that "we need to *develop relevant, acceptable and effective countermeasures* in a timely manner" and fail to mention that these countermeasures are diagnostics, vaccines and medicines, i.e., they can be part of *essential medicines.*

References

ACMA. (2023). 5 Reasons biologics remain expensive. 13 July 2023. https://medicalaffairsspecialist.org/blog/5-reasons-biologics-remain-expensive.

Annett, S. (2021). Pharmaceutical drug development: High drug prices and the hidden role of public funding. *Biologia Futura, 72,* 129–138. https://doi.org/10.1007/s42977-020-00025-5

Driece, R. A., Matsoso, P., et al. (2023). A WHO pandemic instrument: Substantive provisions required to address global shortcomings. *The Lancet, 401.* 29 April 2023. https://www.thelancet.com/action/showPdf?pii=S0140-6736%2823%2900687-6

Even, P., & Debré, B. (2012). Guide de 4 000 médicaments, utiles, inutiles ou dangereux. Cherche Midi (Ed.), Paris.

Le Monde. (1979). Le règne des multinationales, Claire Brisset. 3 January 1979. https://www.lemonde.fr/archives/article/1979/01/03/le-regne-des-multinationales_2787987_1819218.html

Naddaf, M., & Nature Magazine. (2022). $3.5-Million hemophilia gene therapy is world's most expensive drug. 9 December 2022. https://www.scientificamerican.com/article/3-5-million-hemophilia-gene-therapy-is-worlds-most-expensive-drug/.

O'Neill Institute, Foundation for the National Institutes of Health, University of Cape Town. (2023). Emergency Countermeasure Development and Deployment, November 2023. The O'Neill Institute for National and Global Health Law, Foundation for the National Institutes of Health, University of Cape Town. 1 November 2023. https://oneill.law.georgetown.edu/publications/emergency-countermeasure-development-and-deployment/.

Quick, J. D., Hogerzeil, H. V., Velásquez, G., & Rago, L. (2002). Twenty-five years of essential medicines. *Bulletin of the World Health Organization, 80*(11), 913–914. World Health Organization. https://iris.who.int/handle/10665/268659

Swissinfo. (2019). How can a drug cost 2.1 million dollars? 29 May 2019. https://www.swissinfo.ch/eng/business/explainer_how-can-a-drug-cost-2-1-million/44996728

Velásquez, G. (1991). Tiers-monde magazine, PUF (Presses Universitaires de France), Tome XXXII—N0. 127, July–September 1991.

WHO. (1990). The use of essential drugs (1989) - TRS 796. WHO Technical Report Series, No. 796. Geneva: World Health Organization, 1990. https://www.who.int/publications/i/item/9241207965.

WHO. (2023a). The selection and use of essential medicines 2023: Executive summary of the report of the 24th WHO Expert Committee on Selection and Use of Essential Medicines 24–28 April 2023. Geneva: World Health Organization; 2023 (WHO/MHP/HPS/EML/2023.01). https://iris.who.int/bitstream/handle/10665/371291/WHO-MHP-HPS-EML-2023.01-eng.pdf?sequence=1.

WHO. (2023b). WHO model lists of essential medicines. July 2023. https://www.who.int/groups/expert-committee-on-selection-and-use-of-essential-medicines/essential-medicines-lists.

WHO Division of Drug Management and Policies. (1988). Global medium-term programme: Programme 12.2, essential drugs and vaccines, eighth general programme of work covering the period 1990–1995. World Health Organization EDV/MTP/88.1. https://iris.who.int/handle/10665/62717.

Chapter 7
The Announcement of the United States' Withdrawal From the WHO: "Shooting Oneself in the Foot..."

7.1 Introduction

In July 2020, President Donald Trump made one of the most controversial announcements of his first presidency: the United States would withdraw from the World Health Organization (WHO). This decision came in the midst of the COVID-19 pandemic, a global health crisis that highlighted the need for international cooperation. By signalling his intention to leave the WHO, Trump not only distanced the US from a crucial institution, but also undermined global efforts to combat pandemics, protect public health and safeguard the health of the most vulnerable populations around the world.

Fortunately, what he announced in 2020 did not come to pass because the administrative process could not be completed before the end of his term. When Democrat Joe Biden became President, he reversed the decision before the process initiated by his predecessor was completed.

Now, at the start of his second term, Trump has again announced that the US will formally leave the WHO in 2025. Leaving the WHO is a financial blow to the organization, as many have pointed out, but it is much more than that.

7.2 US Presence in the WHO

The United States has been the largest financial contributor to the WHO for 30 years and its contribution represents today about 15 percent of the total budget WHO (6.8 billion US dollars by 2024–2025) (EURACTIV, 2025). In the late 1990s a resolution of the World Health Assembly, led by the United States, approved the freezing the budget of the WHO with a "zero real growth" policy, which lasted for 30 years (Velasquez, 2024).

© The Author(s), under exclusive license to Springer Nature Switzerland AG 2025
G. Velásquez, *Negotiating Global Health Policies*, SpringerBriefs in Public Health, https://doi.org/10.1007/978-3-031-99847-8_7

The original rule for the WHO budget was that each country gave a financial contribution according to certain parameters such as GDP and number of inhabitants, and that each country participated equally in the decisions. This is the general policy of the United Nations "one country one vote" (United Nations, 2018).

The decision to freeze the WHO budget more than 30 years ago prompted some industrialized countries to increase their contributions with the so-called "voluntary contributions", generally earmarked for specific programmes selected by these countries. Voluntary contributions from a small group of industrialized countries and the private sector now account for 84 percent of the total WHO budget (Velásquez, 2024). In the case of the United States, their overall contribution for 2024–2025 was 958 million US$, of which about US$ 260 million is the contribution mandatory to the regular budget (Statista, 2025).

The exaggerated financial weight of the voluntary contributions of the United States, as well as of other industrialized countries, complicates the democratic functioning of the organization, because the large donor countries (of voluntary contributions) have a strong control over the programmes and priorities of the organization and the policy of the United Nations—"one country one vote"—is thus almost impossible to apply. There are many global public health issues on which the United States is constantly threatening to use its power of veto. Thus, in many cases, its presence translates into excessive control of one member state within an organization that has 194 members.

As French historians Jean-Paul Gaudillière and Christophe Gradmann put it in an article for *Le Monde*, "Donald Trump's attacks on the World Health Organization are not simply a strategy to deconstruct multilateralism. They are linked to differences of opinion about the organisation's governance, mission and practices" (Le Monde, 2025).

7.3   A Blow to the Multilateral System

The US withdrawal from the WHO undermines the very principles of multilateralism and cooperation that have been fundamental to the post-World War II international order. Global health challenges demand collective action and, by distancing itself from the WHO, the US is signalling that it is unwilling to collaborate with other countries to solve common problems. This is a dangerous precedent that could have far-reaching consequences, not only for cooperation in public health, but also for the prevention and management of future health crises.

While multilateralism is a fundamental principle of international cooperation, the WHO has witnessed how the US Government, in recent years, far from playing the rules of multilateralism, has been constantly exerting bilateral pressures within this multilateral body.

The multilateral system of cooperation seeks to solve global problems through consensus among member states, avoiding the hegemony of dominant actors and promoting greater equity in decision-making. The multilateral forum provided by the WHO is supposed to give countries, regardless of their size or power, the opportunity to influence the global agenda and participate in the creation of international norms that protect all. This unfortunately has not been always the case. We can take the example of the negotiations on a binding international treaty for the prevention of future pandemics over the past 3 years, where the US Government has systematically opposed anything that affects its commercial interests such as those of the pharmaceutical or food industries, even if the proposals in the treaty were in the interests of safeguarding the health of everyone in the world.

Seen from this perspective, Trump's recent decision to withdraw from the WHO is somewhat strange, as it deprives them of a way of defending their own interests.

Indeed, one might also wonder, even in financial terms, which of the two stands to lose more, the WHO or the United States—or to be more precise, the US pharmaceutical industry? In 2021, Pfizer reported $36 billion in revenue from the sale of the COVID-19 vaccines alone, making it the world's best-selling pharmaceutical product that year. Was it not the WHO that facilitated the sharing of data that enabled the development of COVID-19 vaccines? Was it not the WHO that facilitated and promoted the mass use of vaccines?

7.4   A False Justification, and a Reckless Decision for Global Health

Trump's justification for withdrawing from the WHO was based on his bogus argument that the organization is ineffective and overly influenced by China. He frequently claimed that the WHO had failed to act swiftly and transparently at the onset of the COVID-19 pandemic, and that it had become "China-centric" (The White House, 2025).

While it is "healthy" to question the actions of any international organization, including the WHO, Trump's decision to abandon the WHO is reckless, counterproductive and, why not say it, irresponsible. The World Health Organization has been central to responding to global health emergencies for more than seven decades. Its work in the fight against diseases such as smallpox, polio, Ebola and HIV/AIDS, or the binding international convention against tobacco use, has saved millions of lives.

The COVID-19 pandemic is a clear example of why global health cooperation is vital. In an interconnected world, no country is an island when it comes to infectious diseases. A virus that spreads in one country can quickly become a global threat, as we experienced with COVID-19. The WHO has provided essential guidance on testing, treatment, vaccine development and public health strategies. Its global health expertise is irreplaceable, and its leadership is needed now more than ever. With the United States' withdrawal from the WHO, the American administration is sending the message that the United States is not willing to contribute to collective efforts to protect humanity from pandemics, setting back global health initiatives by years, if not decades.

The WHO also provides technical assistance to countries that lack the infrastructure or resources to mount effective responses to health crises. By withdrawing, the US would be abandoning those who depend on international cooperation and support. Trump's decision demonstrates a worrying indifference to the health and well-being of millions of people around the world, especially in developing countries that depend in some way on WHO collaboration for critical health interventions.

The United States' withdrawal from the World Health Organization (WHO) will have a serious impact on various aspects of global health, but the United States will itself be directly affected. Indeed, a key issue is the impact that withdrawal will have on health research. There are currently 72 WHO Collaborating Centres in the United States which draw on information collected by the WHO in its 194 Member States (WHO, 2025a). Depriving these collaborating centres of global information would affect health research activities and the development of technologies, medicines and vaccines by US industry.

The Lancet, the renowned medical journal, strongly criticized the move, warning that Trump's withdrawal, by reducing scientific cooperation with collaborating centres, will negatively affect medical research, international cooperation and access to essential health services. *The Lancet* noted that the US exit represents "sweeping and damaging attack on the health of the American people and those dependent on US foreign assistance" (The Lancet, 2025).

7.5   Conclusion

Donald Trump's announcement to withdraw from the WHO in 2025 is a reckless decision with far-reaching consequences. It represents a short-sighted and self-defeating approach to global health that puts both the United States and the world at risk. In an era of interconnected challenges, the United States cannot afford to disengage from the global health system. Abandoning this organization at a time when the world faces numerous current and emerging health threats is a grave mistake, where the American president may be "shooting himself in the foot" as the saying goes.

The other 193 WHO member countries should be vigilant to ensure that this announcement does not become a form of blackmail, demanding changes and reforms that only protect the commercial interests of the United States instead of common global health issues.

It is to be expected, as it was already the case during Trump's first term, that the international community will mobilize to compensate for the financial shortfall that this decision may entail. As Michel Kazatchkine says: "The time has come for Europe to distance itself and offer new leadership in place of that abandoned by a former ally that has become unpredictable, if not hostile" (Flahault et al., 2025).

Why not propose a tax on soft drinks, ask Flahault, Calmy and Kazatchkine: "Europe could try to finance the loss of the US contribution to the WHO by introducing a special tax on certain American services and goods, such as soft drinks and ultra-processed foods. A response that would be useful for the health of the public" (Flahault et al., 2025).

Some of the reflections and decisions that will fall to the WHO Secretariat in Geneva and to the member countries to offset this very serious financial decision will include the need to redefine priorities, reduce non-essential operational costs (the Director proposed, for example, drastically reducing travel), and even reviewing the quota of US personnel in the organization. This quota is based on the financial contribution of each country to the organization's budget. Perhaps this crisis would also be an opportunity to reflect on the number of WHO staff at the Secretariat in Geneva (2400 people) (WHO (2025b), while in comparison, the World Trade Organization (WTO) Secretariat in Geneva, to give just one example, employs 620 people (WTO, 2025).

The necessity to strengthen this multilateral agency in the health sector does not make any doubt, for the sake of global health, and thus it is essential that member states unite and find ways of maintaining a strong WHO and counteract this incoherent decision by the current US Administration.

References

EURACTIV. (2025). L'OMS se prépare à réduire son budget après le retrait des Etats-Unis. 3 Feb. 2025. https://www.euractiv.fr/section/sante/news/loms-se-prepare-a-reduire-son-budget-apres-le-retrait-des-etats-unis/.

Flahault, A., Calmy, A., & Kazatchkine, M. (2025). Pour un nouveau leadership en santé mondiale, Le Temps, 16 février 2025. https://www.letemps.ch/opinions/pour-un-nouveau-leadership-en-sante-mondiale?srsltid=AfmBOopMl3yNwYCbE8D1dQV0xIlEVS2YDfEnIIaccF0ncwPCVObwYLE6.

Le Monde (2025). L'Organisation mondiale de la santé déstabilisée par le retrait américain. 21 January 2025. .https://www.lemonde.fr/planete/article/2025/01/21/l-organisation-mondiale-de-la-sante-destabilisee-par-le-retrait-americain-de-l-accord-de-paris_6508506_3244.html?lmd_medium=al&lmd_campaign=envoye-par-appli&lmd_creation=ios&lmd_source=whatsapp.

Statista. (2025). Total U.S. contributions to the World Health Organization (WHO) from 2016–2017 to 2024–2025, by type. https://www.statista.com/statistics/1552800/total-us-contributions-to-who-by-type/#:~:text=In%202024%2D2025%2C%20the%20United,for%20around%20698%20million%20dollars.

The Lancet. (2025). American chaos: Standing up for health and medicine. *The Lancet,* *405*(10477), 439. 8 February 2025. https://www.thelancet.com/journals/lancet/article/PIIS0140-6736(25)00237-5/fulltext.

The White House. (2025). Presidential executive order. Withdrawing the United States from the World Health Organization. 20 January 2025. https://www.whitehouse.gov/presidential-actions/2025/01/withdrawing-the-united-states-from-the-worldhealth-organization/.

United Nations. (2018). 6 things to know about the General Assembly as UN heads into high level week. https://news.un.org/en/story/2018/09/1019842.

Velasquez, G. (2024). Los retos de futuras pandemias: entre la política y la ciencia. Editiones IB de F, Buenos Aires, (p. 55).

WHO. (2025a). WHO Collaborating Centres. Global database. https://apps.who.int/whocc/List.aspx?USZdN9B/p/yKUq4QHE2keA==

WHO. (2025b). Geneva headquarters. https://www.who.int/about/structure.

WTO. (2025). Overview of the WTO Secretariat. https://www.wto.org/english/thewto_e/secre_e/intro_e.htm.

Chapter 8
Final Remarks and Possible Way Forward

Future pandemics are inevitable, due to many causes that we do not address in this book—social inequalities, increasing difficulties of access to health for all, climatic or geopolitical changes. This book is intended to contribute to the reflections underway at the World Health Organization to prepare more appropriate responses to these future pandemics.

To prepare appropriate responses to future global health challenges in the area of access to medicines, current challenges and possible future scenarios were discussed in Chap. 2. Three scenarios seem conceivable: a continuation of the current status quo, with a weakened World Health Organization; an increasing shift of decisions on global health into the hands of the G7; and the development of regional solutions.

Given the inability of the multilateral system to adopt global solutions, regional initiatives and solutions could offer more appropriate solutions. These could include the regional manufacture of vaccines and medical supplies, the creation of regional medicines agencies with health standards that promote regional health and production (the Medicines Agency for Latin America and the Caribbean—AMLAC—proposed by certain Latin American countries, or the African Medicines Agency, currently being set up), as well as a regional approach to intellectual property rules, the use of flexibilities in the Agreement on Trade-Related Aspects of Intellectual Property Rights (TRIPS), cooperation and the strengthening of South–South cooperation. This new regional dynamic could at the same time enable a return to more equitable multilateral relations in the future, to the benefit and well-being of all.

Support for healthcare in developing countries, and in particular access to medicines in the event of pandemics, depends in part on development cooperation funds. These funds represent only a small part of the investments made in developing countries to support their healthcare systems. However, not all of these funds in support of health in the South go directly to developing countries, but are channelled largely through public–private consortia and other entities such as the Global Fund, CEPI, COVAX, the WHO Foundation and the World Bank FIF. Almost half of the

G. Velásquez, *Negotiating Global Health Policies*, SpringerBriefs in Public Health, https://doi.org/10.1007/978-3-031-99847-8_8

aid goes to buy medicines and vaccines produced in a small group of developed countries, which are virtually the same as those supplying these public–private consortia.

The impasse in the multilateral global health arena lies partly in the origin of its funding, as discussed in Chap. 3. The management of COVID-19 by CEPI, COVAX, and the recent creation of the WHO Foundation and the FIF at the World Bank, indicate that the industrialized countries prefer and seek to impose global health management governed by public–private consortia designed by these countries. For its part, the WHO—which has been authorized to symbolically increase its public budget—could act only as a non-voting observer, providing technical assistance to the public–private consortia that will take the decisions.

The rhetoric says that the WHO coordinates and governs, but in practice it confines itself to giving technical recommendations and observing the decision-making process in bodies where it is merely an observer. The role of the "WHO Foundation", which has never been approved by the WHO governing bodies, is ambiguous, and the mechanisms for avoiding conflicts of interest are not sufficiently clear.

Will the G7 and, after it, the G20 take the reins and impose their vision of global health management?

Recent international speeches, the World Health Assembly 2022, the G7 and G20 reports, all speak of strengthening the role of the WHO, as a lesson from the COVID-19 epidemic. It is in this sense that we can understand the decision of the World Health Assembly to gradually increase the regular public budget to 50 percent of public contributions by 2028–2029. However, the total increase in contributions to the organization's regular public budget would only represent an increase of 1.2 billion dollars, which could be compared with perplexity to the billions that the entities and mechanisms referred to above will manage or aspire to manage.

We have seen how international solidarity has failed to guarantee access to vaccines, diagnostics and treatments. The COVID-19 crisis has prompted the international community to reflect on the need for a binding international treaty on pandemics. At the time when the pandemic was still raging, Russia launched a senseless and costly war against Ukraine, and the Atlantic Alliance embarked on an arms race that risks diverting urgently needed healthcare funding to the purchase of arms. Real preparation for future pandemics clearly requires the strengthening of the public health sector, including the WHO, and the funding that is currently dispersed among a multitude of entities and mechanisms that fragment the global health system instead of making it more coherent and robust.

As for the binding treaty aimed at preventing future pandemics, which has been under negotiation at the WHO for almost 3 years, it must be recognized that it is far from adequately responding to the challenges raised by the COVID-19 crisis.

If new negotiations are to take place, as decided by the World Health Assembly in 2024, the first thing to do would be to analyse, identify and acknowledge the reasons why the negotiations failed within the timeframe set. It is not simply a question of continuing negotiations to "refine the current draft". The document should be substantially redrafted to contain legally binding measures to address the issue of access to research & development and to the technologies needed to produce essential medicines for future pandemics.

The research, development and marketing of medicines in the United States of America, the European Union and Japan are highly profitable industries where commerce and profit take precedence over the well-being and health of citizens. The regional approach that Colombia, Cuba and Mexico (Acapulco Declaration); and Argentina, Brazil, Chile, Colombia, Cuba and Mexico (Bogotá meeting on regulatory convergence) want to adopt today is a new way of looking at drug R&D, manufacturing and marketing.

The challenge we face today is to ensure that health comes first, that medicines are not simply commodities but public goods that serve to protect and restore people's health. The creation of regional agencies, such as the medicines agencies in Latin America and Africa, could meet this challenge. In a market of 500 million people, as is the case in Latin America, the public good represented by medicines could also contribute financially to the region's economy.

The concept of "essential medicines" launched by the WHO in 1977 in response to the proliferation of pharmaceutical products on the markets of many countries is undoubtedly one of the greatest achievements of this organization in its history. Based on this concept, most countries in the world have developed national medicines policies, theories on medicines as public goods have been developed and many of us have argued that access to essential medicines is a citizen's right.

The crisis caused by the COVID-19 pandemic, which many of us thought would lead us to rethink a better world, has paradoxically been a step backwards in some areas. The debate on access to diagnostics, vaccines and treatments, which for 50 years have been included in the concept of essential medicines, has led some people to develop ambiguous terms that have little to do with public health, such as "medical countermeasures" or "health countermeasures". These new terms are closer to commoditized "health products" than to common public goods.

Chapter 6 discusses how the fundamental concept of "essential medicines" is seemingly being replaced by the concept of "medical countermeasures" or "health countermeasures". This is an example of how international health negotiations can weaken and undermine the fundamental concepts of public health developed by the WHO and many of its member countries.

Today, essential medicines policies are implemented in most countries within their healthcare institutions or systems. Why this change? The disorganization of global health: the privatization of the WHO, the involvement of the G7 and G20 in global health, the emergence of a multitude of new players, the tendency and pressure from developed countries to leave everything in the hands of public–private entities?

In this new scenario, and probably partly because of it, the pharmaceutical products and new therapeutics of the last 10 years are entering the markets but are inaccessible even to many developed countries' health systems. We are therefore going to repeat the injustice of 20 years ago, when the first antiretroviral drugs for AIDS arrived, once again leaving the vast majority of the world's population living in developing countries excluded from the progress and discoveries of health sciences.

Preparing for future pandemics requires us to ask this fundamental question: how can the public interest, the defence of common public goods and the protection of human rights be safeguarded in the prevention, preparation and response to current and future pandemics?

Appendix: Recent South Centre Research Papers on Public Health

No.	Date	Title	Author
96	August 2019	Antivirales de acción directa para la Hepatitis C: evolución de los criterios de patentabilidad y su impacto en la salud pública en Colombia	Francisco A. Rossi B. y Claudia M. Vargas P.
100	December 2019	Medicines and Intellectual Property: 10 Years of the WHO Global Strategy	Germán Velásquez
101	December 2019	Second Medical Use Patents—Legal Treatment and Public Health Issues	Clara Ducimetière
103	February 2020	Eighteen Years After Doha: An Analysis of the Use of Public Health TRIPS Flexibilities in Africa	Yousuf A Vawda & Bonginkosi Shozi
104	March 2020	Antimicrobial Resistance: Examining the Environment as Part of the One Health Approach	Mirza Alas
105	March 2020	Intersección entre competencia y patentes: hacia un ejercicio pro-competitivo de los derechos de patente en el sector farmacéutico	María Juliana Rodríguez Gómez
107	April 2020	Guide for the Granting of Compulsory Licenses and Government Use of Pharmaceutical Patents	Carlos M. Correa
108	April 2020	Public Health and Plain Packaging of Tobacco: An Intellectual Property Perspective	Thamara Romero
112	June 2020	La judicialización del derecho a la salud	Silvina Andrea Bracamonte and José Luis Cassinerio

(continued)

© The Author(s), under exclusive license to Springer Nature Switzerland AG 2025
G. Velásquez, *Negotiating Global Health Policies*, SpringerBriefs in Public Health, https://doi.org/10.1007/978-3-031-99847-8

(continued)

No.	Date	Title	Author
113	June 2020	La evolución de la jurisprudencia en materia de salud en Argentina	Silvina Andrea Bracamonte and José Luis Cassinerio
114	June 2020	Equitable Access to COVID-19 Related Health Technologies: A Global Priority	Zeleke Temesgen Boru
116	August 2020	The TRIPS Agreement Article 73 Security Exceptions and the COVID-19 Pandemic	Frederick Abbott
118	September 2020	Re-thinking Global and Local Manufacturing of Medical Products After COVID-19	Germán Velásquez
119	October 2020	TRIPS Flexibilities on Patent Enforcement: Lessons from Some Developed Countries Relating to Pharmaceutical Patent Protection	Joshua D. Sarnoff
120	October 2020	Patent Analysis for Medicines and Biotherapeutics in Trials to Treat COVID-19	Srividya Ravi
121	November 2020	The World Health Organization Reforms in the Time of COVID-19	Germán Velásquez
124	November 2020	Practical Implications of 'Vaccine Nationalism': A Short-Sighted and Risky Approach in Response to COVID-19	Muhammad Zaheer Abbas
125	December 2020	Designing Pro-Health Competition Policies in Developing Countries	Vitor Henrique Pinto Ido
126	December 2020	How Civil Society Action can Contribute to Combating Antimicrobial Resistance	Mirza Alas Portillo
129	March 2021	The TRIPS waiver proposal: an urgent measure to expand access to the COVID-19 vaccines	Henrique Zeferino de Menezes
133	August 2021	Malaria and Dengue: Understanding two infectious diseases affecting developing countries and their link to climate change	Mirza Alas
134	September 2021	Restructuring the Global Vaccine Industry	Felix Lobo
135	September 2021	Implementation of a TRIPS Waiver for Health Technologies and Products for COVID-19: Preventing Claims Under Free Trade and Investment Agreements	Carlos M. Correa, Nirmalya Syam and Daniel Uribe
136	September 2021	Canada's Political Choices Restrain Vaccine Equity: The Bolivia-Biolysis Case	Muhammad Zaheer Abbas
140	November 2021	Del SIDA al COVID-19: La OMS ante las crisis sanitarias globales	Germán Velásquez
141	November 2021	Utilising Public Health Flexibilities in the Era of COVID-19: An Analysis of Intellectual Property Regulation in the OAPI and MENA Regions	Yousuf A Vawda and Bonginkosi Shozi

(continued)

(continued)

No.	Date	Title	Author
142	4 January 2022	Competition Law and Access to Medicines: Lessons from Brazilian Regulation and Practice	Matheus Z. Falcão, Mariana Gondo and Ana Carolina Navarrete
143	11 January 2022	Direito Brasileiro da Concorrência e Acesso à Saúde no Brasil: Preços Exploratórios no Setor de Medicamentos	Bruno Braz de Castro
144	27 January 2022	A TRIPS-COVID Waiver and Overlapping Commitments to Protect Intellectual Property Rights Under International IP and Investment Agreements	Henning Grosse Ruse-Khan and Federica Paddeu
145	9 February 2022	The Right to Health in Pharmaceutical Patent Disputes	Emmanuel Kolawole Oke
146	16 February 2022	A Review of WTO Disputes on TRIPS: Implications for Use of Flexibilities for Public Health	Nirmalya Syam
147	28 February 2022	Can Negotiations at the World Health Organization Lead to a Just Framework for the Prevention, Preparedness and Response to Pandemics as Global Public Goods?	Viviana Muñoz Tellez
147	28 February 2022	Can negotiations within the World Health Organization lead to a fair framework for the prevention, preparedness and response to pandemics as a global public good?	Viviana Muñoz Tellez
147	28 February 2022	¿Podrán las negociaciones en la organización mundial de la salud resultar en un marco justo para la prevención, la preparación y la respuesta ante pandemias como bienes públicos globales?	Viviana Muñoz Tellez
152	21 April 2022	An Examination of Selected Public Health Exceptions in Asian Patent Laws	Kiyoshi Adachi
153	26 April 2022	Patent Analysis for Medicines and Biotherapeutics in Trials to Treat COVID-19	Srividya Ravi
154	9 May 2022	COVID-19 Vaccines as Global Public Goods: Between life and profit	Katiuska King Mantilla and César Carranza Barona
158	15 June 2022	Twenty Years After Doha: An Analysis of the Use of the TRIPS Agreement's Public Health Flexibilities in India	Muhammad Zaheer Abbas
143	11 January 2022	Brazilian Competition Law and Access to Health in Brazil: Exploitative Pricing in the Pharmaceutical Sector	Bruno Braz de Castro
166	6 October 2022	Lessons From India's Implementation of Doha Declaration on TRIPS and Public Health	Nanditta Batra

(continued)

(continued)

No.	Date	Title	Author
168	28 October 2022	TRIPS Flexibilities and Access to Medicines: An Evaluation of Barriers to Employing Compulsory Licenses for Patented Pharmaceuticals at the WTO	Anna S.Y. Wong, Clarke B. Cole, Jillian C. Kohler
169	8 November 2022	The WTO TRIPS Decision on COVID-19 Vaccines: What is Needed to Implement it?	Carlos M. Correa and Nirmalya Syam
170	17 November 2022	Left on Our Own: COVID-19, TRIPS-Plus Free Trade Agreements, and the Doha Declaration on TRIPS and Public Health	Melissa Omino and Joanna Kahumbu
171	29 November 2022	Pautas para el Examen de Solicitudes de Patentes Relacionadas con Productos Farmacéuticos	Carlos M Correa
171	31 January 2022	Guidelines for the examination of patent applications relating to pharmaceutical products	Carlos M Correa
173	7 February 2023	Analysis of COVID-Related Patents for Antibodies and Vaccines	Kausalya Santhanam
174	13 February 2023	Leading and Coordinating Global Health: Strengthening the World Health Organization	Nirmalya Syam
175	22 March 2023	Experiencias internacionales sobre la concesión de licencias obligatorias por razones de salud pública	Catalina de la Puente, Gastón Palopoli, Constanza Silvestrini, Juan Correa
176	29 March 2023	De dónde viene y a dónde va el financiamiento para la salud	Germán Velásquez
178	22 May 2023	A Response to COVID-19 and Beyond: Expanding African Capacity in Vaccine Production	Carlos M. Correa
179	14 July 2023	Reinvigorating the Non-Aligned Movement for the Post-COVID-19 Era	Yuefen Li, Daniel Uribe and Danish
180	9 August 2023	Neglected Dimension of the Inventive Step as Applied to Pharmaceutical and Biotechnological Products: The case of Sri Lanka's patent law	Ruwan Fernando
184	15 September 2023	Promoting Jordan's Use of Compulsory Licensing During the Pandemic	Laila Barqawi
186	14 November 2023	Patentamiento de anticuerpos monoclonales. The case of Argentina	Juan Correa, Catalina de la Puente, Ramiro Picasso y Constanza Silvestrini
188	7 December 2023	The Intersection Between Intellectual Property, Public Health and Access to Climate-Related Technologies	Lívia Regina Batista
190	24 January 2024	Implementing the Doha Declaration in OAPI Legislation: Do Transition Periods Matter?	Patrick Juvet Lowé Gnintedem

(continued)

(continued)

No.	Date	Title	Author
191	25 January 2024	TRIPS Waiver Decision for Equitable Access to Medical Countermeasures in the Pandemic: COVID-19 Diagnostics and Therapeutics	Nirmalya Syam and Muhammad Zaheer Abbas, PhD
192	30 January 2024	Pautas para el examen de patentes sobre anticuerpos monoclonales	Juan Correa, Catalina de la Puente, Ramiro Picasso y Constanza Silvestrini
193	2 February 2024	Desafíos actuales y posibles escenarios futuros de la salud mundial	Germán Velásquez
194	15 February 2024	Implementation of TRIPS Flexibilities and Injunctions: A Case Study of India	Shirin Syed
195	6 March 2024	Régimen de licencias obligatorias y uso público no comercial en Argentina	Juan Ignacio Correa
196	19 April 2024	Licencias obligatorias para exportación: operacionalización en el orden jurídico argentino	Valentina Delich
197	28 May 2024	Compulsory Licensing as a Remedy Against Excessive Pricing of Life-Saving	Behrang Kianzad
201	27 June 2024	Antimicrobial Resistance: Optimizing Antimicrobial Use in Food-Producing Animals	Viviana Munoz Tellez
202	28 June 2024	Constraints to and Prospects for Sustainable Livestock Sector Practices in Argentina with Emphasis on Antimicrobial Usage	David Oseguera Montiel
203	11 July 2024	The Vaccine Industry After the COVID-19 Pandemic: An International Perspective	Felix Lobo
204	24 July 2024	Negotiating Health and Autonomy: Data Exclusivity, Healthcare Policies and Access to Pharmaceutical Innovations	Henrique Zeferino De Menezes, Julia Paranhos, Ricardo Lobato Torres, Luciana Correia Borges, Daniela De Santana Falcão and Gustavo Soares Felix Lima
206	28 August 2024	Equity and Pandemic Preparedness: Navigating the 2024 Amendments to the International Health Regulations	Nirmalya Syam
208	10 September 2024	Catalyzing Policy Action to Address Antimicrobial Resistance: Next Steps for Global Governance	Anthony D. So
209	25 September 2024	AMR in Aquaculture: Enhancing Indian Shrimp Exports through Sustainable Practices and Reduced Antimicrobial Usage	Robin Paul

Index

B
Binding treaty against pandemics, 51–52, 78
BRICS, 5, 11–14

C
Coalition for epidemic preparedness
        innovations (CEPI), 5, 7, 38,
        42, 77, 78
COVAX, 5, 7, 11, 18, 33, 38, 42, 54, 77, 78
COVID-19, 2, 6, 11, 21, 25, 26, 38, 41, 42, 48,
        49, 53, 54, 60, 73, 78
COVID-19 crisis, 7, 11, 18, 39, 47, 52, 78
COVID-19 pandemic, 7, 8, 10, 15, 19–21, 25,
        32, 33, 38, 42, 47, 48, 50, 63, 67,
        71, 73, 79

E
Essential medicines, 3, 19, 33, 52, 60, 61,
        63–68, 78, 79

F
Future pandemics, 2, 3, 6, 15, 42, 48, 49,
        51–52, 55, 73, 77, 78, 80

G
G20, 5, 7, 9, 11–14, 38, 42, 78, 79
Global health, 1–3, 5–21, 26, 28, 30, 31, 33,
        35, 36, 39, 40, 42, 47–50, 53, 67,
        71–75, 77–79

Global health financing, 25–42
The Group of Seven (G7), 1, 2, 5–7, 11–14,
        18, 19, 42, 77–79
Group of 77 + China, 5, 14–15, 50

H
Health financing, 1, 10, 21, 32

I
Intergovernmental Negotiating Body (INB), 2,
        6, 48, 49, 51, 52, 67, 68
International cooperation, 15, 50, 71, 72, 74
International Council for Harmonisation
        (ICH), 59, 60
International Health Regulation (IHR), 2,
        6, 53–55
International Health Regulations (IHRs), 6, 19,
        20, 47–55, 59
International Monetary Fund (IMF), 5,
        7–10, 13
International negotiations, 3
International solidarity, 26, 42, 50, 78

L
Latin America and the Caribbean, 15, 58, 77

M
Medical countermeasures, 3, 15, 52, 63–68, 79
Multilateralism, 1, 5, 15, 16, 21, 26, 53, 72

N

Negotiation of international pandemic treaties,
      2, 47–55, 63
Non-aligned countries, 16
North-South relations, 15

O

Official development assistance (ODA) for
      health, 32–33

P

Pharmaceutical policies, 36, 58, 66
Philanthropic organizations, 16
Privatisation of health, 8, 30–32, 79
Public-private partnerships, 7, 12, 25

R

Regional drug regulatory agencies, 57, 58, 61

S

Standards for drug regulation, 59

U

UN Global Compact, 29
US Administration, 75

W

WHO and UN agencies (World Health
      Organization and United
      Nations), 1, 5, 6, 12,
      14, 17, 19, 26, 27,
      30, 72
WHO budget, 1–2, 28, 35, 38, 72
World Bank, 1, 5, 7–10, 13, 16, 18,
      30–33, 35, 41, 42, 77, 78
World Health Assembly (WHA), 2, 15,
      16, 27, 31, 32, 37, 39–42,
      48, 49, 51, 53–55, 59, 67,
      71, 78
World Health Organization (WHO), 1, 6,
      26, 47, 58, 63,
      71, 77
World Intellectual Property
      Organization (WIPO), 5, 37
World Trade Organization (WTO), 5, 26,
      37, 67, 75

The manufacturer's authorised representative in the EU is Springer
Nature Customer Service Centre GmbH, Europaplatz 3, 69115 Heidelberg,
Germany. If you have any concerns regarding our products, please
contact ProductSafety@springernature.com

Printed and bound by CPI Group (UK) Ltd, Croydon, CR0 4YY

28/04/2026

02098544-0002